THE WAI'ANAE BOOK OF HAWAIIAN HEALTH

No Ka Wai'anae Diet

Haku 'ia na Mililani Allen
March 16, 1992

E Kūkulu kumuhana nā po'e Hawai'i
Pull together Hawaiian people

Hemolele i ka hihia
Free the entanglements

Ho'okuakahi i ka pōhaku
Clear the way of stones

E 'ai i ke kalo
Eat the taro

Ke kino o Hāloa
The body of Hāloa

E inu i ka wai
Drink the water

Ka wai ola o Kāne
The waters of life of Kāne

© WCCHC 1991

E kūkulu kumuhana nā po'e Hawai'i
Pull together Hawaiian people

Ho'ola ke kino
Heal the body

Hui 'ia mākou i ka ola kino.
We join together in health.

This book is dedicated to our kupuna,
who have taught us; and to our kamalii
who will carry on,

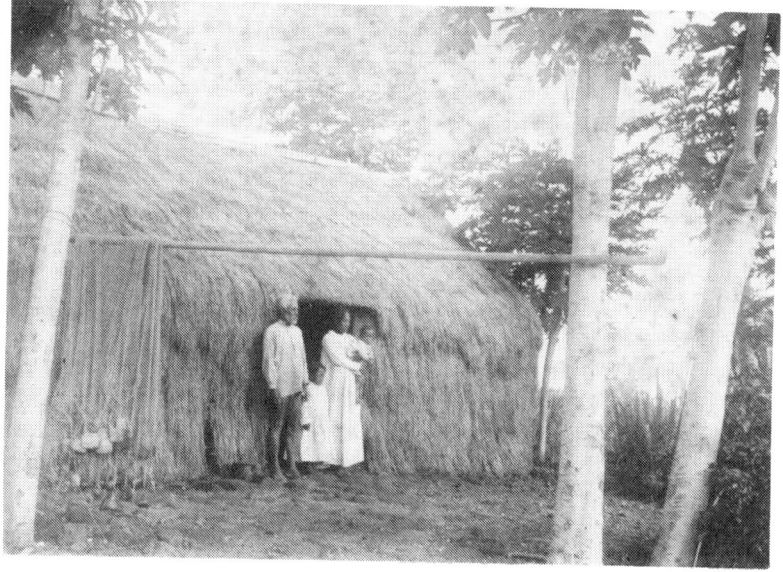

A Hawaiian Family in Front of a Grass House. Circa, 1890.
Courtesy of Bishop Museum

and to the Memory
of Edward Kaonohiokala Aikala
(1941-1991)

Editors:
Terry Shintani, M.D., M.P.H. and Claire Hughes, M.S., R.D.

Contributing Authors:
Sheila Beckham, M.P.H., R.D.; Kekuni Blaisdell, M.D.; Midge Eli; Eric Enos; Claire Hughes, M.S., R.D.; Kamaki Kanahele; Helen Kanawaliwali O'Connor; Terry Shintani, M.D., M.P.H.

Advisory Committee:
Noa Emmett Aluli, M.D.; Sheila Beckham, M.P.H., R.D.; Kekuni Blaisdell, M.D.; Ho'oipo DeCambra; Frenchy DeSoto; Eric Enos; Flo Kahaleua; Claire Hughes, M.S., R.D.; Kamaki Kanahele; Germaine Keliikoa; Helen Kanawaliwali O'Connor; Terry Shintani, M.D., M.P.H.; and Frances Sydow, Ph.D.

Faculty:
Mililani Allen; Kekuni Blaisdell, M.D.; Agnes Cope; Claire Hughes, M.S., R.D.; Kamaki Kanahele; Louise Kong; Lisa Laronal; and Katherine Maunakea.

Group I Staff for the Wai'anae Diet Program:
Midge Eli; Flo Kahaleua; Helen Kanawaliwali O'Connor; Musu Maneafaiga; Sheila Beckham, M.P.H., R.D.; and Frankie Paragoso

Group I Participants:
Edward Aikala, Lovey Aina, Nani Bolton, Scott Bush, Eli Carter, Agnes Cope, Ho'oipo DeCambra, Frenchy DeSoto, Fred Eli, Midge Eli, Eric Enos, Vernon Gomes, Black Ho'ohuli, Leina Ho'ohuli, Jerry Iaea, Keli'i Kahele, Kamaki Kanahele, Bernard Maunakea, Karen Maunakea, Robin Maunakea, and Oliver Willingham

Cover Art:
Ka Pu'uwai o Ka Po'e "The Heart of the People" by Kawena Young

Artwork and Publishing:
Eric Uptegrove, Eric Enos, Sue Teehan, Jean Curry, and Jan Foster

TABLE OF CONTENTS

Acknowledgments iv
Special Acknowledgments v
Preface vii
Introduction 1
History 5
Health 9
    Early Disease 10
    Modern Disease 11
Politics 13
Economics 15
Principles 17
    Principles of Attitudinal Healing 20
Spirit *(Mana)* 21
    Spiritual Recipe 23
Mind *('Ano'Ano)* 25
    'Ano'Ano: The Seed 26
    Recipe For The Mind 27
Emotion *(Aloha)* 29
    Aloha 30
    Emotional Recipe 31
Body *(Kino)* 33
    Kino 34
    Pono (Balance, Harmony) 35
    Restoring Pono 36
    Physical Activity 36
    Physical Recipe 38
The Wai'anae Diet 39
    Getting Started with the Wai'anae Diet ... 41
    The Wai'anae Diet Menu 44
    Foods and Recipes 45
The Wai'anae Diet Transition Program 71
    Transition Diet Menu 72
    Transition Recipes 74
Results of the Wai'anae Diet 87
Comments From Program Participants 103
Beginnings 117
Bibliography 119

ACKNOWLEDGMENTS

The contributions of many organizations and individuals have made the Wai'anae Diet Program a reality, and to them we extend our sincere gratitude.

- We acknowledge and thank the Board of Directors of the Waianae Coast Comprehensive Health Center (WCCHC) who supported the creation and implementation of this program, and the staff members who invested many hours to its development.
- Kahumana Farm provides the site for the program and generously donated their kitchen, dining facilities, and staff time.
- Honolulu Poi Company was generous with donations of the main staple of the diet, delicious poi.
- The 'Opelu Project and Ka'ala Farm, organizations who strive to restore the ahupua'a concept, provided resources on farming and growing taro, as well as other cultural topics which are depicted in their book "From Then To Now. A Manual for Doing Things Hawaiian Style."
- Na Pu'uwai provided the example of their pioneering effort of the Moloka'i Diet Study, and the technical assistance of Helen O'Connor.
- Claire Hughes, nutritionist at the University of Hawaii School of Public Health, assisted in all phases of development and initiation of the Program.
- Historical photographs of The Bishop Museum are an important part of the Program, providing us visual information about the past; and "Voices on the Wind," by Palani Vaughn inspired us to pursue the physical profiles of the past.
- OHA, K108 radio's "Nutrition and You" program, the Honolulu Star Bulletin, Honolulu Magazine, KITV, KHON, and KGMB have all generously provided information to the community about the diet.
- The James and Abigail Campbell Foundation helped by providing funds for the publication of the first edition of this book.
- The Robert E. Black Memorial Trust provided funds to repeat the program with long-term follow-up.
- The Honorable Governor John Waihe'e wholeheartedly provided his moral support to the Program.
- And finally, our warmest mahalo to the participants of the first Wai'anae Diet Program who are proponents, teachers, and role models. These Hawaiians continue to sow the seeds of the Wai'anae Diet Program so that greater numbers of Hawaiians may benefit.

SPECIAL ACKNOWLEDGMENTS

To Moloka'i

We would like to express our sincerest appreciation to Na Pu'uwai, a Native Hawaiian health association on Moloka'i that sponsored "The Molokai Diet Study: Ho'oke Ai" in 1987. In that study, ten Native Hawaiians demonstrated the value of the Native Hawaiian diet in lowering high serum cholesterol and triglycerides which are both risk factors for heart disease. Mahalo nui loa for your pioneering efforts and for your assistance and support in helping to make the Wai'anae Diet Program a success.

To Kahumana Farm and Community Center

We would also like to express our special gratitude to Kahumana Farm and Community Center which provided free of charge the dining hall, cooking facilities, and some of the staff support, without which the Wai'anae Diet Program could not have occurred. The Kahumana Farm and Community Center continues to pursue programs for the health and well being of people on the Wai'anae Coast.

To HPC Foods (Honolulu Poi Company)

Special acknowledgement also goes to HPC Foods who from the very outset has supported us through three projects with donations of poi.

To Robert E. Black Memorial Trust

The first organization to financially support the program was the Robert E. Black Memorial Trust. They provided support for WDP Phase II in the third year of the project.

To James and Abigail Campbell Foundation

The James and Abigail Campbell Foundation has helped by providing us funding for the first printing of this book and is providing funds for the cookbook that is scheduled to be published in early 1993.

To Office of Hawaiian Affairs (OHA)

In 1992, OHA has graciously provided us with the funding to continue the program in Waianae and to develop the program. In addition, the funding is intended to help start similar programs on the neighbor islands and to other communities on Oahu.

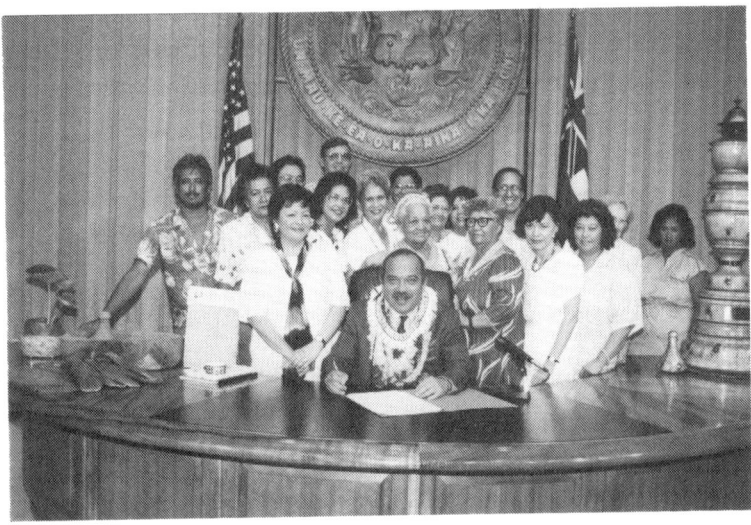

The Honorable Governor John Waihe'e signing the Proclamation of Taro Awareness Month in recognition of the Wai'anae Diet Program and two Taro festivals taking place in September, 1989. *(There is a Wai'anae Diet plate lunch and bag lunch to the right of the Governor on the table.)*

PREFACE

The purpose of this book is to help you to improve your health and your life as a whole, and to help to do the same for all the Hawaiian people. In the spirit of "lōkahi," this book was a joint effort of various members of the Waiʻanae Coast community, in conjunction with the generous help of individuals from "town" and from Molokaʻi.

Hawaiian health is a critical issue today because in Hawaiʻi, "the healthiest state in the union," Native Hawaiians have the worst health in the nation. This is in sharp contrast to the excellent health that the Hawaiians had in pre-Western contact times, before 1778 when Captain Cook arrived. Today, Hawaiians have the highest rates of heart disease, cancer, stroke and diabetes in the state. Over 70% of all Hawaiians die of these diseases, and all of these diseases are diet-related. This is the reason why the main focus of this book is on diet.

> **Let us Hawaiians be in the front leading all the people together.**
> – Jay Landis

Why should a book about Hawaiian health come from Wai'anae? First of all, the Wai'anae coast has the largest concentration of Hawaiian people in the state. According to the 1980 U.S. Census, 56% of the people in Nanakuli and 34% of the Wai'anae people are Hawaiian. Second of all, the Wai'anae coast has the poorest economic conditions in the state and some of the poorest health. Yet, Wai'anae is rich in Hawaiian tradition and in human resources and spirit.

> **It is important for us to utilize our kupuna' mana'o because after they're gone, who will teach us?**
> – Richard Kalolo'okalani Keaulana

This book and the Wai'anae Diet Program are efforts to make use of this richness to reverse an epidemic of diet-related deaths among the Hawaiian people, both in this community and across the state.

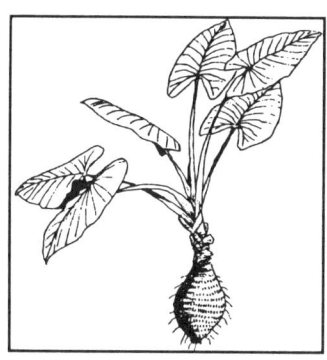

INTRODUCTION

Aloha. By picking up this book, you have taken the first step towards a commitment to make a difference in your own life. If you want to look and feel better – this book is for you. In this book are ideas that can help you to change your life for the better. You have also taken an important step towards making a positive difference in the lives of people around you. We hope this book will plant the seeds that will enable you to influence the health of your family, friends, and ultimately all the Hawaiian people.

What's In This Book For You?

In this little book, the WAI'ANAE BOOK OF HAWAIIAN HEALTH, you will learn why ancient Hawaiians were among the healthiest people on earth. With this in mind, we present steps to help restore, maintain, and maximize your health. You will learn four steps to long-term weight loss. You will be provided with some simple Hawaiian methods for helping you make your dreams a reality. Perhaps, most important of all, you will be invited to participate in a great movement to restore the good health of all the Hawaiian people.

While food is the major focus of this book, we would like to emphasize that this book is one that touches on all aspects of the person, including the physical, mental, emotional, and spiritual. It will look at the whole person in the context of his or her environment, including the social, political, and economic status. The reason for this is that "ola lōkahi" is a guiding principle of this program. That is, that all things and all people are connected. In the same way, the whole person is connected in all his or her aspects. Health is not related just to diet. It includes physical activity, positive attitude, harmonious relationships with others and all things around you, and a faith in a power beyond ourselves.

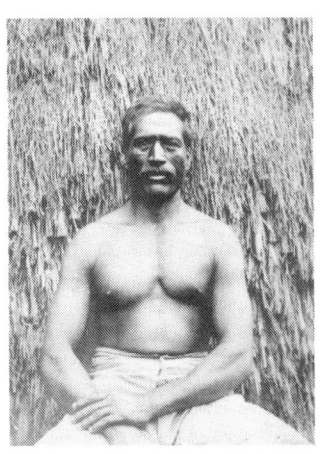 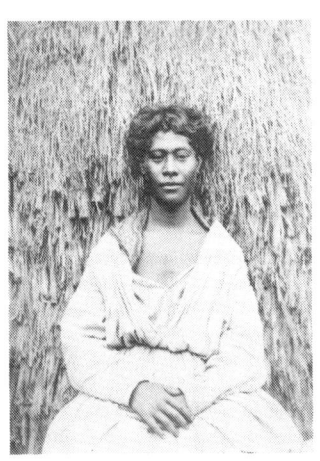

Hawaiian Man and Hawaiian Woman, circa 1890
Bishop Museum Visual Arts Collection

Preview of This Book

In the first section of this book, we will discuss how the Hawaiian people were among the healthiest, most energetic and active people on earth. We will explore some of the basic principles that helped to support this healthy lifestyle. Then we will point out how Western influence has changed the cultural, political and socioeconomic circumstances that have strongly influenced the health of the Hawaiian people. In the latter sections of this book, the spiritual, mental, emotional and physical aspects of health are discussed. The Wai'anae Diet Program is presented in the last section of this book so that you can take some steps to start to create your own health.

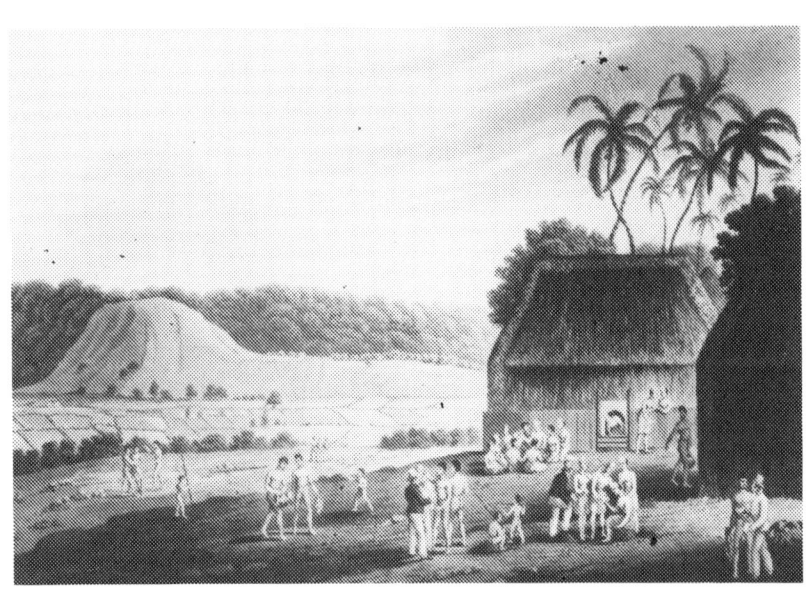

Village of Macacoupou, Owhyee
Heddington, Pub. 1814, *Courtesty of Bishop Museum*

HISTORY

In the beginning, God created the heavens and the earth. In Hawaiian mythology, as documented in the ancient Hawaiian creation chant, He Kumulipo, sky father was known as "Wakea" and mother earth was known as "Papa." Through the mating of Wakea and Papa all things came to be. It started with the tiny creatures of the ocean, from the coral polyps, to the plants and other creatures of the sea and land, and finally to man.

Because all things share the same "parents," Papa and Wakea, all things are connected and living. The connecting force was known as "mana" or "life force." This understanding was the basis of the concept of "ola lōkahi" . . . ola meaning "life," and lōkahi meaning "oneness." The words *ola lōkahi* taken together mean "oneness of life" or "oneness of the universe."

The common people are . . . of a thin rather than full habit.

– Stewart 1825

In other words, everything in the universe is living and connected with each other.

The first born child of Papa and Wakea named Haloa was stillborn. He was buried in the earth with great sorrow. But, because of the great love of Papa and Wakea, there was great

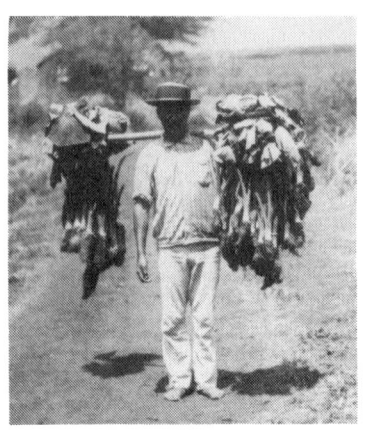

Taro Vendor
Courtesy of Bishop Museum

mana in this child, and out of the body of this child grew kalo *(taro)*, which proliferated throughout Hawai'i. Because of this great mana found in kalo, it provided life force to support and nurture the lives of the descendants of Papa and Wakea. While all foods have mana and provide some life force to those who consume them, kalo, in Hawaiian tradition, has special mana.

Since everything is connected and everything is living, it was important to be "pono," or in harmony or balance with everything. This includes harmony with the land, the fauna, the flora, the food, oneself, and all other people including one's ancestors. It is a fundamental understanding that loss of pono is the cause of illness. This included the loss of harmony with the land, or the food, or some pilikia *(trouble)* with another person. Of course, there was a special reverence for food, in particular kalo, because of its mana; all foods were appreciated.

These foods . . . these sources of mana . . . were abundant and could be found from the tops of the mountain peaks to the lowlands, to the bottom of the ocean. Anyone could live a happy and industrious life on an ahupua'a because all of his or her needs could be provided for on such a region, including fruit from the mountains, water from the streams, kalo from the lowlands, and fish from the ocean.

As a result, the Hawaiian people flourished over the years. They reached a maximum population of about one million at the time of the arrival of the first Westerners with Captain Cook in 1778.

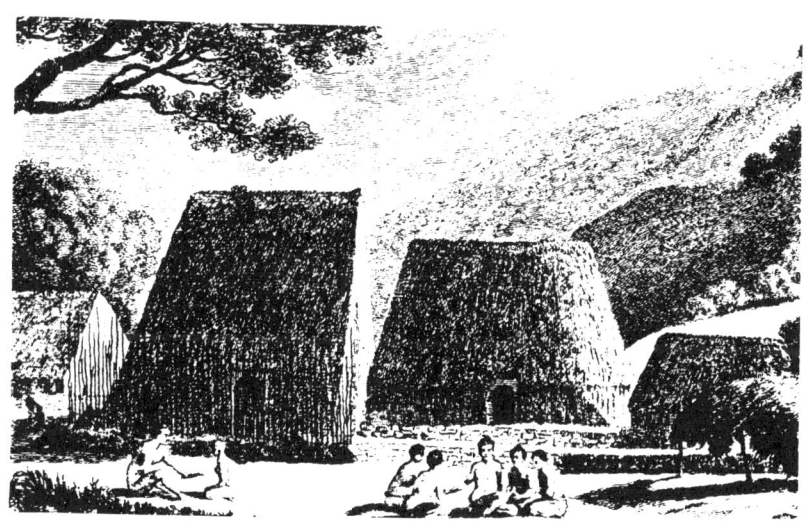

Courtesy of Bishop Museum

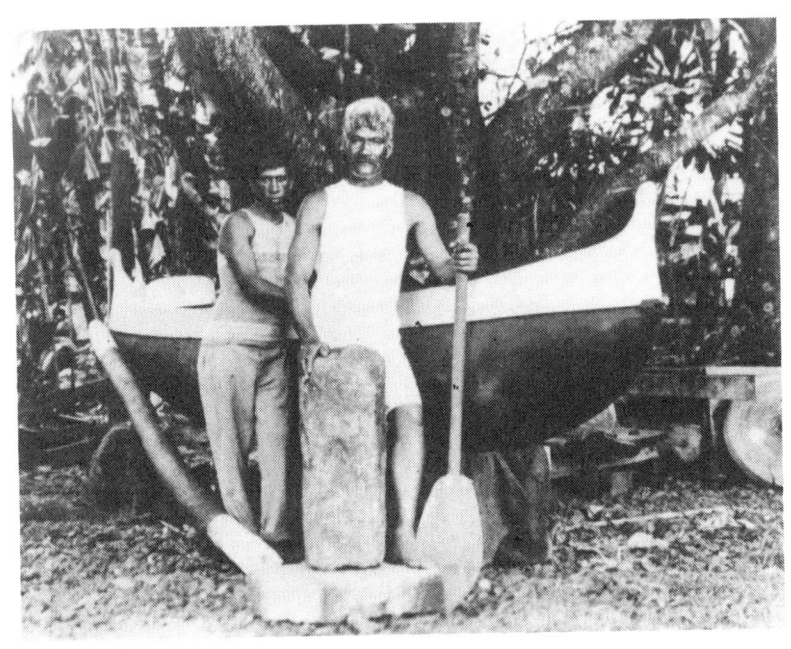

Two Men at Makaokūikalani Stone
Theodore Kelsey, *Courtesy of Bishop Museum*

HEALTH

The Hawaiian of the past was thin and strong rather than overweight. Let us repeat that . . . they were **thin** rather than overweight *(see photo, p. 5)*. In other words, their natural status was to be slim. This is in contrast to the commonly held belief that Hawaiians were naturally obese. If you have doubts about the truth of this statement, just look at the pictures of ancient Hawaiians in this book and ask yourself, "Where are the overweight Hawaiians?"

The Hawaiian people were tall, "above the middle stature, . . . graceful and . . . stately." They were attractive and healthy. This was the conclusion of this early observer in times soon after Western contact. Hawaiian people today have it in them to be this way, if we return to some of the ways of our kupuna.

> **The natives are in general above the middle stature, well formed with fine muscular limbs; their gait graceful and sometimes stately.**
> – Ellis 1832

> The natives of these islands are, in general, above the middle size and well made; they walk very gracefully, run nimbly and are capable of bearing great fatigue.
> – Capt. James King, 1779

In addition to being taller than average, the Hawaiian people were ". . . capable of bearing great fatigue." In other words, they were energetic, active and strong. This energy and hard working nature was a reflection of their excellent health. A high level of physical activity was a normal part of Hawaiian life.

Early Disease

With exposure to Western influence, the population began to decline. The main cause at first was infectious disease. Within the first century of Western contact, literally hundreds of thousands of Hawaiians died of diseases such as syphilis, gonorrhea, smallpox, mumps, and measles. In 1804, there was a terrible plague that wiped out over half the population of Hawai'i. It was so swift that people would be stricken in the morning and be dead by nightfall.

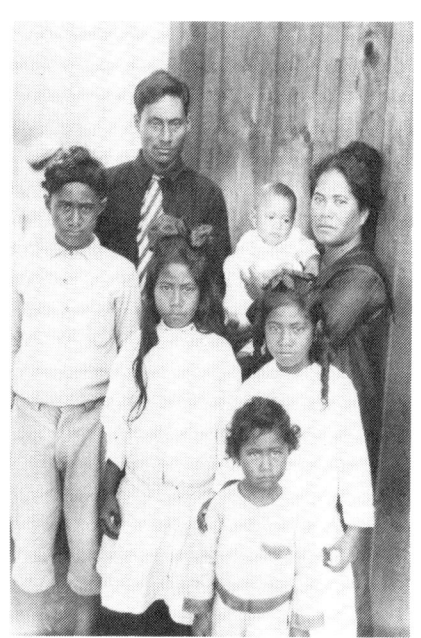

Pōaha Family
Puko'o, Moloka'i, 1921
Courtesy of Bishop Museum

Modern Disease

After much of the Hawaiian population met its demise through infectious disease, and after vaccines and sanitation began to control these illnesses, a new epidemic has been claiming the lives of the Hawaiian people. This epidemic is diet-related disease. The change to a more westernized diet and away from the traditional Hawaiian diet has brought with it very high rates of heart disease, cancer, strokes and diabetes. In fact, the rates of death from these diet-related diseases for pure Hawaiians are the highest in the nation (see page 92).

POLITICS

In the 1848, the Mahele created private ownership of land. Less than 20% of the common people received less than 1% of the land. The ahupua'a system was abandoned. Thus, a major foundation of Hawaiian life was destroyed.

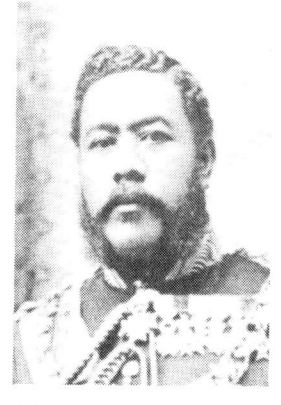

King David Kalakaua 1881, *Courtesy of Bishop Museum*

The power of the Hawaiians was stolen from them at gunpoint in 1887. In that year, a group of powerful, non-Hawaiian businessmen forced King David Kalakaua to sign a new constitution, under threat of militiamen with rifles and bayonets.

This new constitution called the "bayonet" constitution vested most of the power in the house of lords which was made up of only landowners. Since very few Hawaiians owned land at this time, this virtually disenfranchised the Hawaiian people and gave all the power to non-Hawaiians. This loss of control over their own affairs hastened the downward spiral of the Hawaiians' economic, social, and cultural condition.

> **A sad thing was when a lot of Hawaiians lost their lands . . . When the old folks passed away, no one bothered about the land.**
> — James Robinson Holt III

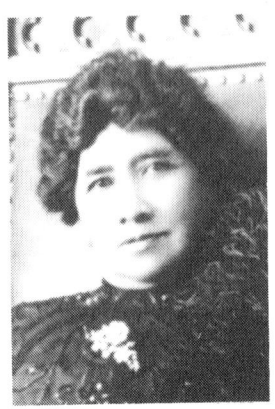

Queen Lili'uokalani
1897, *Courtesy of Bishop Museum*

The last Hawaiian ruler of the Hawaiian kingdom was Queen Lili'uokalani, who succeeded her brother, King David Kalakaua, when he died in 1891. She tried to regain the power of the monarchy and the control of Hawai'i by Hawaiians, by proposing a new constitution. In 1893, businessmen backed by U.S. armed forces compelled her to yield her authority, and a provision government was established.

In 1894, Queen Lili'uokalani was arrested and tried, and forced to renounce all claims to the throne. With the overthrow of the Hawaiian monarchy, and U.S. annexation in 1898, Hawaiians were politically disenfranchised and no longer controlled their lands.

ECONOMICS

Since that time, economic conditions for the Hawaiian people have remained poor and, accordingly, their health has suffered. The Westernization of their diet has played a major role in this poor health. Today, Hawai'i is the healthiest state in the union. In sharp contrast, the health of the Hawaiian people is among the worst in the nation.

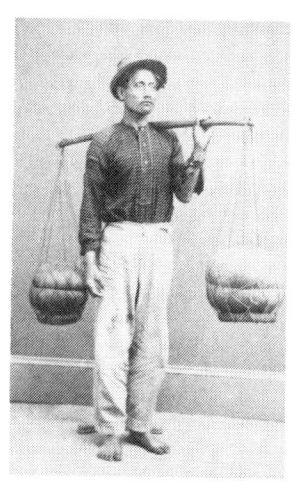

Hawaiian Poi Dealer, *Courtesy of Bishop Museum*

The largest concentration of Hawaiians is on the Wai'anae Coast, with roughly 16,000 Hawaiians living there. The poorest economic conditions are found there, as well as the worst health. For this reason, it is most appropriate to begin the Wai'anae Diet Program on the Wai'anae Coast.

OLA LŌKAHI: A Hawaiian Key To Health

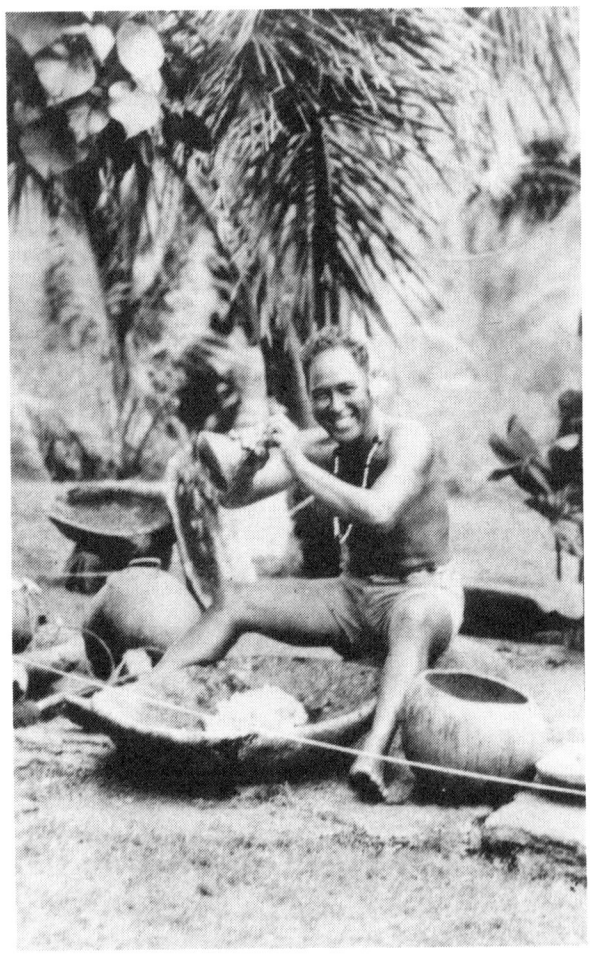

Pounding Poi, 1932
Courtesy of Bishop Museum

PRINCIPLES - By Kekuni Blaisdell, M.D.

Because of common parentage from Papa and Wakea, the kanaka maoli *(as Native Hawaiians called themselves)* considered himself lōkahi *(united)* with all in the cosmos from the beginning and forever.

In spite of the prevailing spirituality, all in the Hawaiian cosmos was natural. There was nothing "supernatural" in the Western sense. Events could and were influenced by all of the numerous forces in the material and spiritual cosmos, favorable and adverse, from the past as well as in the present. These included the individual kanaka's thoughts and attitudes, as well as his actions.

Palua *(dualism)* of complementary opposites was also recognized, such as sky and earth, day and night, sun and moon, male and female, right and left, hot and cold, fire and water, material and spiritual, health and illness, good and evil, and life and death.

Pono, or proper order or harmony of these interacting, cyclic and opposing forces required conscious effort, including each individual kanaka's participation.

Kapu *(sacred restricting taboo)*, established by the kahuna *(priest specialists)*, sanctioned by the ruling ali'i and enforced by all, was society's way of preserving pono for the common good. For the kapu fostered self-discipline and responsibility in personal hygiene, health-promotion, illness-prevention, public sanitation and respect for the sacredness of nature.

Imbalance of mana or loss of pono accounted for misfortune, such as illness.

While there was collective lōkahi and interdependence with self – na'au *(gut, as the seat of thought and feelings)*, kino *(body)*, 'uhane *(personal spirit lodged within the skull)*, wailua *(dream soul which occasionally wandered)* – and others, such as 'ohana *(family)* including 'aumakua, kahuna, and ali'i, nevertheless, individual self-reliance was expected.

Each child was a precious pua *(flower)* assuring perpetuation of the race. Adults, of course, were the providers. And the elderly were esteemed. Death after a meaningful life were welcomed as a reuniting with one's kupuna *(ancestors)* in the eternal spiritual realm, with completion of a recurring cycle of rebirth and transfiguration into kinolau or reincarnation into other human forms. Thus, the kanaka considered himself part of a continuum with his kupuna before him, all of his present 'ohana and nature about him during his physical existence or ola *(life)* on earth, and with his offspring and succeeding generations after him. An individual alone without these relationships was "unthinkable."

These relationships were promoted by frequent informal, favorable thoughts and spiritual communication with himself, others and all of nature, punctuated by daily, formal rituals to maintain pono or soundness of personal kino *(body)*, beauty and grace, skills, and social, economic and psychic security. Pono with others and with nature assured mau ke ea o ka 'aina, maintenance of "the life of the land."

The traditional law of the land was aloha 'aina, or malama 'aina *(love and care for the land)*. That is, since the resources of the 'aina nurtured kanaka maoli, it was the responsibility of kanaka maoli to cherish and care for the 'aina for subsequent generations. Thus, kanaka were stewards, not private owners, of the 'aina. Their subsistence economy required mutual malama. For the fisherman, providing his catch was not only for himself, but for all in the ahupua'a *(sea-to-mountain region)*. Similarly, the taro planter shared his harvest. And the mauka *(upland)* forester supplied wood for his fellow ahupua'a residents.

Conversely, to intentionally harm others or anything in nature, was to harm oneself . . . .

Principles of Attitudinal Healing

1. The essence of our being is love.
2. Health is inner peace. Healing is letting go of fear.
3. Giving and receiving are the same.
4. We can let go of the past and of the future.
5. Now is the only time there is, and each instant is for giving.
6. We can learn to love ourselves and others by forgiving, rather than judging.
7. We can become love-finders rather than fault-finders.
8. We can choose and direct ourselves to be peaceful inside regardless of what is happening outside.
9. We are students and teachers to each other.
10. We can focus on the whole of life, rather than the fragments.
11. Since love is eternal, death need not be viewed as fearful.
12. We can always perceive others as either extending love, or giving a call for help.

Hawaiian principles and teachings are universal. This is demonstrated by the similarity of Hawaiian principles with this list of "Principles of Attitudinal Healing" from the international organization, Center for Attitudinal Healing.

SPIRIT

MANA

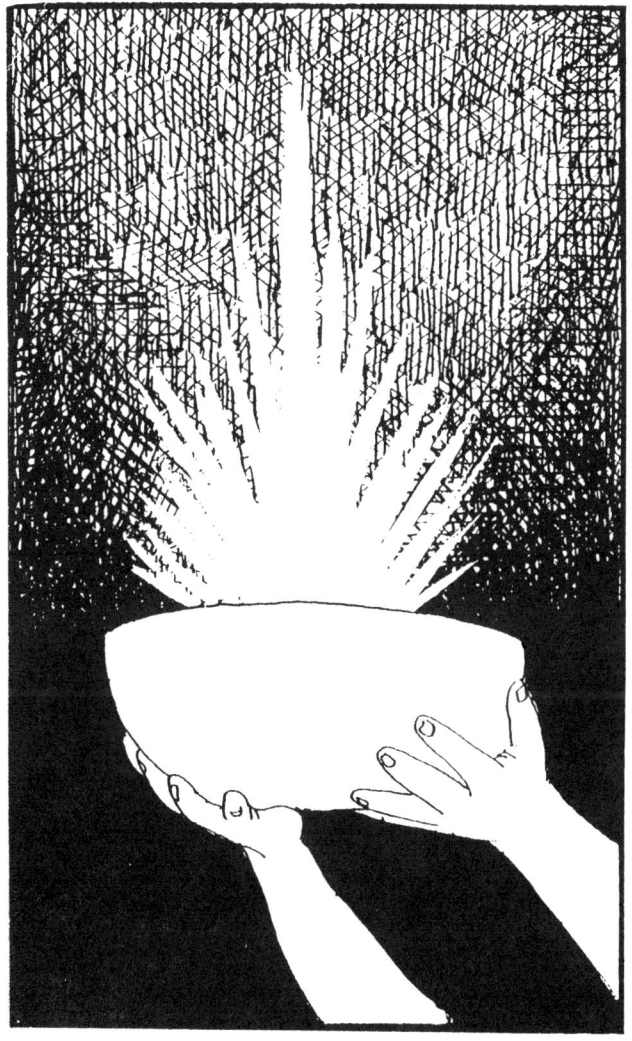

Mana

Mana or special "life force" represents the spiritual side of life. We look at the spiritual side of health first because the ancient Hawaiians were very spiritual. Nothing was considered to be "supernatural," but rather all phenomena were considered to be natural. A life force was in all things, animate and inanimate. It was in human beings, food, plants, trees, animals, the sea and, of course, there was great mana in the land or the 'aina. There was great reverence for all things because of the mana within them.

So in a way, mana can be looked at as the spirit of God within all things. And we should show reverence to all things and all people should have reverence for God. In this way, we maintain "lōkahi" or "unity" with all things and with God. We also help to establish "pono," or a proper relationship with our environment and ourselves. Establishing and maintaining a proper relationship with our environment and the spirit of God in the universe is a major step in maintaining health.

Eating the proper foods is important because life force is present in all foods. Thus food is life-giving, not only from a nutritional standpoint but from a spiritual standpoint as well. Eating food that is closest to its original state would bear the mana from Papa *(earth mother)*. This is one reason that the foods on the Wai'anae Diet Program are not refined and are whole foods. They are similar to the form in which these foods were eaten by the ancient Hawaiians, who had great mana and great health.

Spiritual Recipe

Kahea Ola: To Call to Life

Be aware of the processes of life. As it is in man, so it is in the nature of things. Lessons learned by man from nature allows him to balance a perfect part of life often interrupted by man and his need for assurances and guarantees. For that there is none. All guarantees are only secure if "Ha" *(breath)* is in balance and perfect.

Muʻolau, first phase of budding of the small leaves of a plant.

> *Breathe in long, Mana (give strength) to your breath as in the beginning process of the leaves.*

Muʻolaulani, unfolding of the leaf-budding process.

> *Begin to exhale very gradually spewing forth "Ha," or the life source for growing.*

Muʻoiki, gradually allow the leaf to cease to unfurl.

> *Allow your breathing to subside as its natural pace.*

MIND

'ANO 'ANO

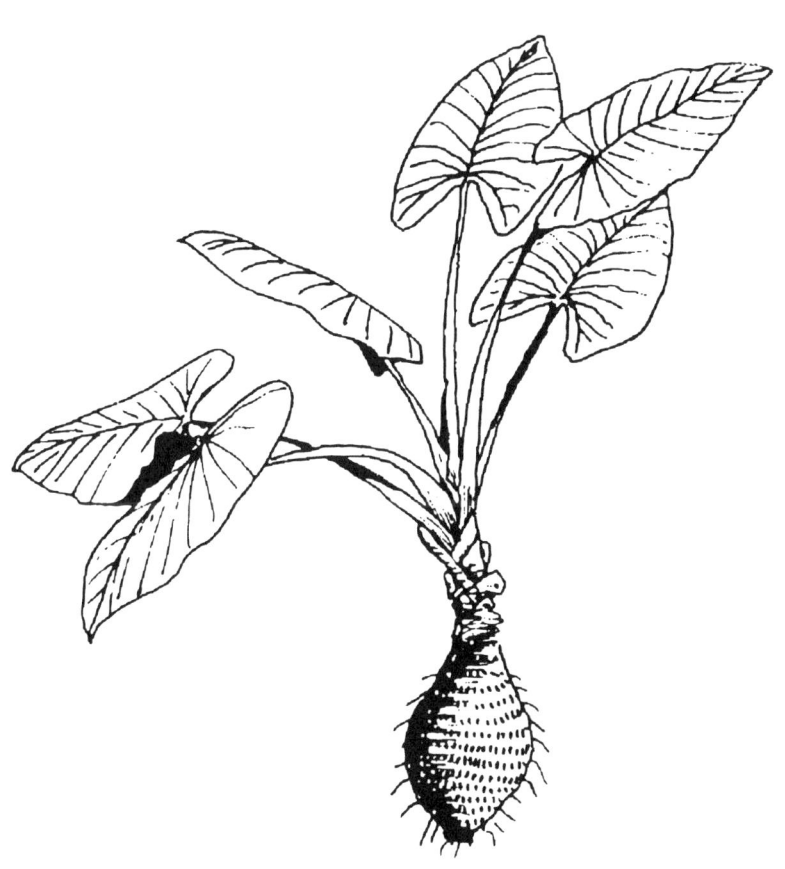

'Ano'Ano: The Seed*

'Ano'Ano *(the seed)* represents the mental aspect of life. This is symbolic of the fact that we create our own reality by what we believe in our mind.

The ancient Hawaiians knew the secret of creating what they wanted on earth. They knew the secret of planting a seed in their minds and nurturing it until it became a reality.

You can achieve anything you want if you know the simple tools that enable you to do this, and if you are willing to pay the price of commitment.

Plant the seed *('Ano'Ano)* in your mind that will blossom into your own health, fulfillment and happiness; and do the same in the minds of all the Hawaiian people.

---

* The title of this section is the same as a book by Kirstin Zambuka published in 1978.

Recipe for the Mind

1. Sit quietly and search your soul to see what it is that you truly desire. Make sure it is what you really want because the universe will give you what you ask.

2. Ask for guidance to ensure that what you want is good for all involved.

3. State clearly in detail the condition you want with words, numbers and data.

4. See this end result in full detail with color, sound and action.

5. Feel what it will be like to have this desired condition.

6. Do not tell others about this seed that you have planted until fruition.

7. Pray for this result each day with the words you have chosen and give gratitude as you visualize the condition as already existing.

EMOTION

ALOHA

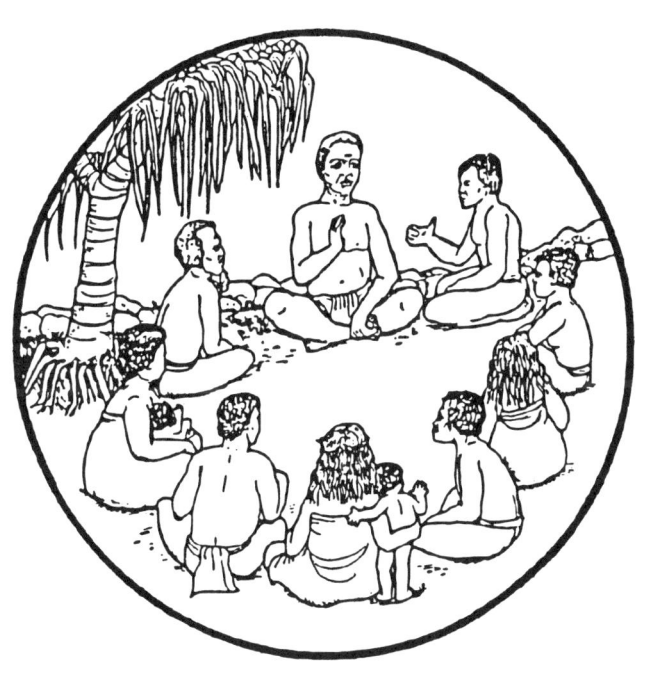

Aloha

Aloha, unconditional love, represents the emotional side of a person, and is the third of four areas which is connected to our health. If we take care of our bodies *(kino)*, we will have emotions that are positive and harmonious. Likewise, if we have positive emotions, such as freely giving love and positive feelings to others, the health of our bodies will be enhanced.

OLA LŌKAHI, in the realm of the emotions of a person, means that we are connected to each other by ALOHA *(love)*. Aloha is at the heart of what it means to be Hawaiian. Freely giving of aloha has long been the hallmark of Hawaiian culture and is a symbol of Hawai'i around the world. This spirit of aloha has fostered a warmth in the Hawaiian culture that is unsurpassed anywhere. A modern representation of the aloha spirit by kupuna Pilahi Paki is as follows:

The Aloha Spirit

- **A** stands for *akahai*, meaning kindness, to be expressed with tenderness.

- **L** stands for *lōkahi*, meaning unity, to be expressed with harmony.

- **O** stands for *'olu'olu*, meaning agreeable, to be expressed with pleasantness.

- **H** stands for *ha'aha'a*, meaning humility, to be expressed with modesty.

- **A** stands for *ahonui*, meaning patience, to be expressed with perseverance.

Emotional Recipe

Mana 'Uhane Aloha: Spiritual Power of Love

Men and Women must again take onto themselves their natural gifts of communicating without words. Too often the spiritual powers of communication are neglected and replaced with the need for verbal satisfaction and gratification. We must utilize this spiritual gift for it controls the secret powers to talk with both plants and animals alike. This inner mana allows for our inner self to come forth with a system of non-verbal communication with powers exceeding those of the verbal world. Aloha Power test samples could include:

- Giving someone a gift that you love for no reason, saying nothing – *feel the Aloha.*

- Touching someone with tender care – *feel the Aloha.*

- Smiling at a person for no reason – *receive it back.*

- Lowering your head in respect to a passing elder – *see the dignity reflected in your Aloha, receive this gift.*

- Doing a good deed without expectation of reward – *feel the Aloha.*

- Making a prideful entrance into an occasion – *feel the dignity.*

BODY

KINO

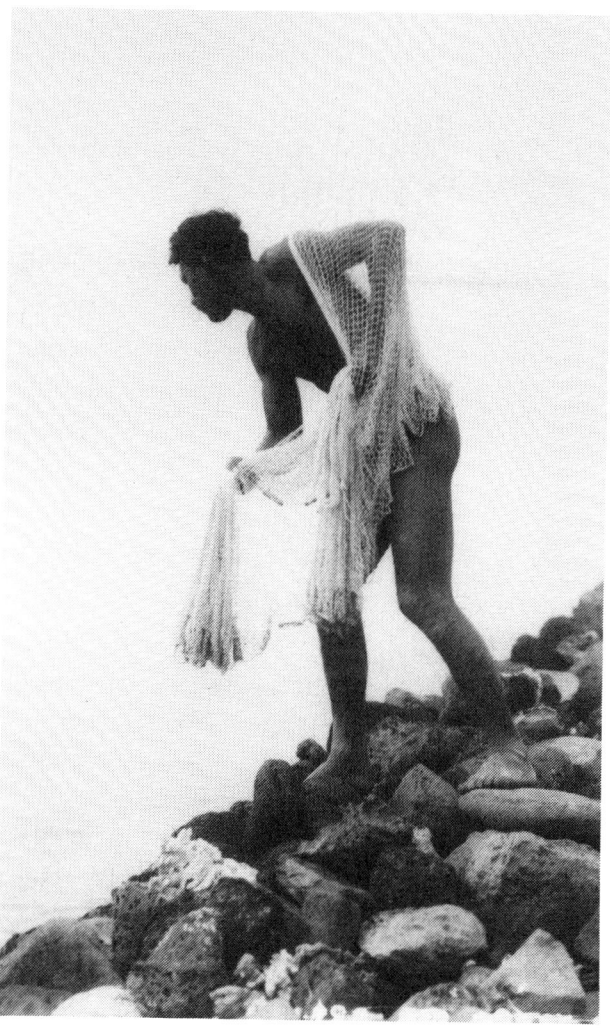

Fisherman Throwing Net
Courtesy of Bishop Museum

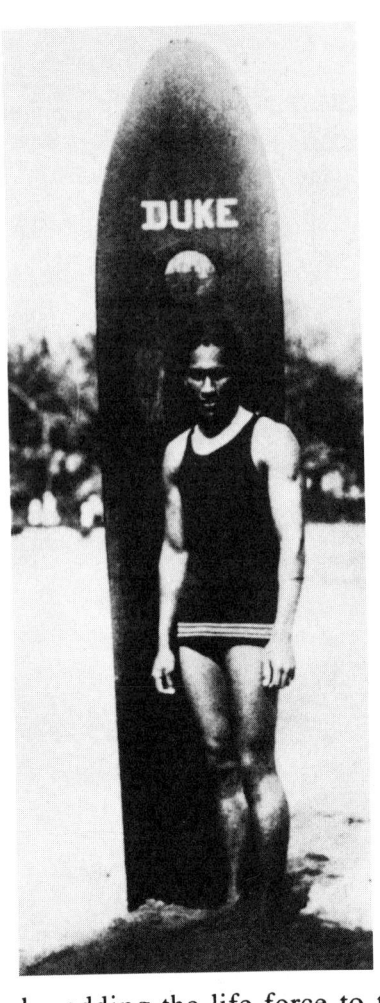

Duke Kahanamoku

Olympic gold medalist in swimming is shown here in Waikiki in 1916.
Courtesy of Bishop Museum

Kino

Kino *(body)* represents the physical side of life. We are connected to our food. This is one way in which the principle of "ola lōkahi" *(oneness with life)* pertains to our bodies. It was a basic understanding of ancient Hawaiians that food, land, water and health were inseparable. It was believed that all foods had a life force, and that eating food was sustaining health by adding the life force to the body.

Kalo *(taro)* was believed to have the greatest life force of all foods because it came from the body of the first-born son of Wakea *(Father heaven)* and Papa *(Mother earth)*. Haloa-naka, as he was named, was buried and out from his body came the kalo *(taro)* plant. Thus, kalo was at the center of the diet and was the chief food of the Hawaiian people. This food was supplemented by other principal foods such as sweet potato, yams, and other foods such as greens, limu *(seaweed)*, fern, fruits and fish.

Pono (Balance, Harmony)

Loss of pono, or loss of balance, was believed to be the cause of all illness. In terms of physical health, loss of pono can be caused by eating the wrong foods. In ancient Hawai'i, the ahupua'a system helped maintain this balance, as this system of land division provided a manner in which people could have access to foods from the highlands down to the sea. In this way, the people were assured of having a balanced diet of a variety of foods.

This belief in the importance of food in the process of healing is demonstrated in the practice of the healing arts of the kahuna lapa'au. When treating the sick, the kahuna would first restrict certain foods. Once the patient agreed to such a restriction, then the kahuna would administer this treatment. (Malo, Hawaiian Antiquities, page 107)

Because of the natural system of ensuring a balanced diet in ancient times, there was not much need for the treatment of diseases that are killing Hawaiians today. There was little obesity. In modern times, the loss of pono in diet is a great problem. Today, obesity is rampant in America and among Hawaiians. In fact, diet-related disease is the number one killer of all Americans. Hawaiians also die at a much greater rate of these diseases than others.

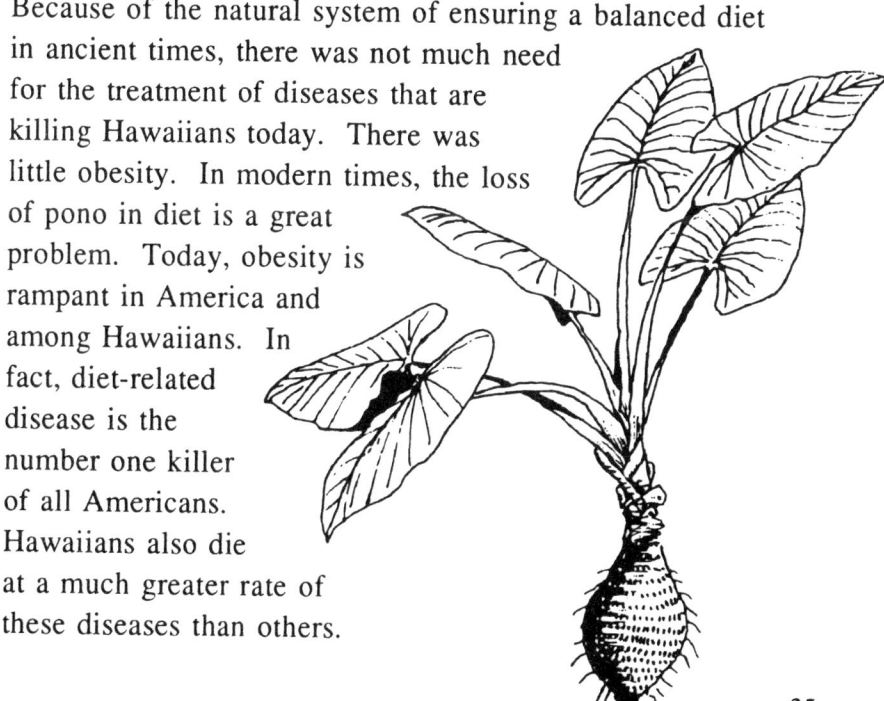

Restoring Pono

One way to restore the health of the Hawaiian people is to restore "pono" in the diet. Because bad diet is the greatest killer of Hawaiians today, the largest section of this book is on food. This is the reason the Waiʻanae Diet Program focuses on restoring "pono" in the diet. One of the basic parts of this diet is to restore the principal food, along with the natural food of the Hawaiians. That is, to revert to taro and poi as the chief food of Hawaiians, mixed with a variety of other foods that were present before Western contact. While this is not practical on a large scale at this time *(because taro is expensive and in short supply)*, there are reasonable modern substitutes that are inexpensive that we can use in the meantime with positive results.

Physical Activity

Establishing "pono" in the "kino" *(body)* also means physical activity. It makes sense that what goes in must go out, and the energy taken in must be balanced by an equal amount going out in the form of physical activity. Physical activity was again a natural part of Hawaiian life. In the *Journal of a Voyage Between China and the Northwestern Coast of America* published by W. Shaler in 1808 (p. 112), an early visitor noted that the Hawaiian people were "the most industrious people I ever saw."

> **... the most industrious people I ever saw.**
> – W. Shaler, 1808

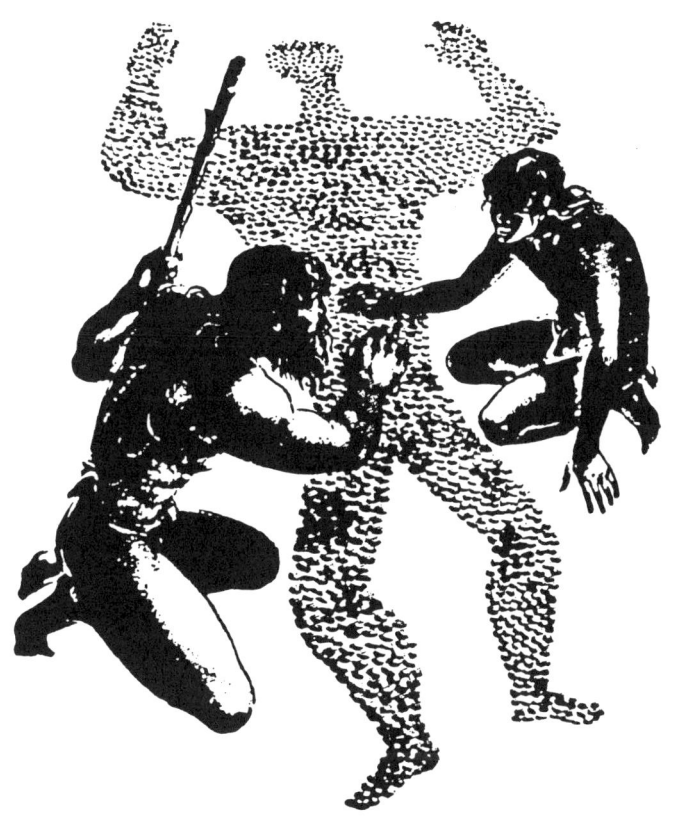

A kahuna lapa'au teaching an apprentice the anatomy of the human form using some 480 white, red, and black pebbles arranged in the shape of a man representing some 280 diseases.

Courtesy Bishop Museum Press

Physical Recipe

Enjoy your physical side each day by exercising daily *(or at least three or four times a week)* for at least 30 to 40 minutes. Walking, swimming, jogging, and aerobics are good examples of what you can do. Try to do it with someone so that it is more fun. If you live on the Wai'anae Coast, then take care of your kino by enjoying the Wai'anae Diet. Call 696-7081 and ask for the Health Education Department for any exercise program that may be available.

- Check with your doctor if you have health problems about the kind of exercises you can do.

- Find an exercise you enjoy and has your doctor's approval.

- Do the exercise(s) at least four times per week for 30 to 40 minutes per day.

- If possible, find a friend to exercise with.

- Follow the Wai'anae Diet Program.

- Share the Wai'anae Diet Program with your friends.

THE WAI'ANAE DIET

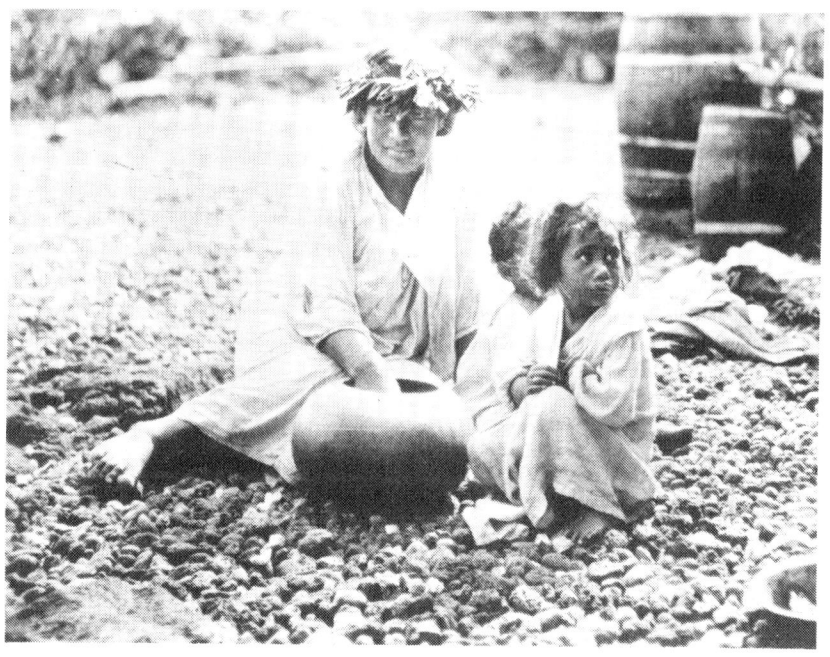

Eating Poi – Lāhainā, Maui, 1901
Courtesy of Bishop Museum

Before You Change Your Diet

This book provides information about health and diet in general and is not to be taken as professional advice for your health problems. If you are seriously ill or on medication, do not change your diet or medications without consulting your physician.

Getting Started With The Wai'anae Diet

Getting started with the Wai'anae Diet can be simple and fun. Before you start, remember that if you have health problems, especially if you are on medication, you must see your physician and get his or her okay, because this diet is so effective that you may need to reduce your medication. Remember that this is not a substitute for medical care.

First, see your doctor if you have health problems or are taking medication.

Second, try to do this diet with a friend or family member, such as your spouse, so that you have some support. If you can attend a Wai'anae Diet presentation, try to do so. You can find out by calling (808) 696-7081 and asking for the Wai'anae Diet Program.

Third, stock your kitchen. Here are some things you may need.

Food

Kalo *(taro)*
Sweet potato
Poi
'Ulu *(breadfruit)* in season
Lu'au leaf – cooked or raw

Limu *(if available)*
Bananas
Fish
Ti leaf *(ki)*
Mamaki tea
Ko'oko'olau tea

Equipment

Pots and Steamer

Fourth, cooking methods includes steaming, baking, broiling, and boiling. Foods were never fried in oils.

Fifth, practice these principles of eating:

a. Express your gratitude before eating and understand that you are connected to the aina through the mana of your food.

b. The main dish is kalo, or poi, or other starch *(such as sweet potato)*, so most of the food you eat should be from this group.

c. Greens are also eaten in large amounts and are unlimited.

d. The fish, fruit, limu and other foods are side dishes.

e. Chicken and wild fowl *(birds)* are eaten less often – usually on special occasions.

f. Pork or other meat is rarely eaten.

g. Salt is added in small amounts at the table after cooking.

h. Eat in an unhurried manner and chew your food.

Sixth, Of course, kalo, poi and other Hawaiian foods are expensive and often in short supply. For meals in which you cannot get the ancient foods, modern equivalents are listed after each section.

Seventh, remember to take care of the spiritual, mental, emotional parts of you by following the daily recipes in this book.

Eighth, share – tell others about your new way of life and about this book so that many Hawaiians may restore their health as quickly as possible. This is your diet and your way of living, so become a teacher.

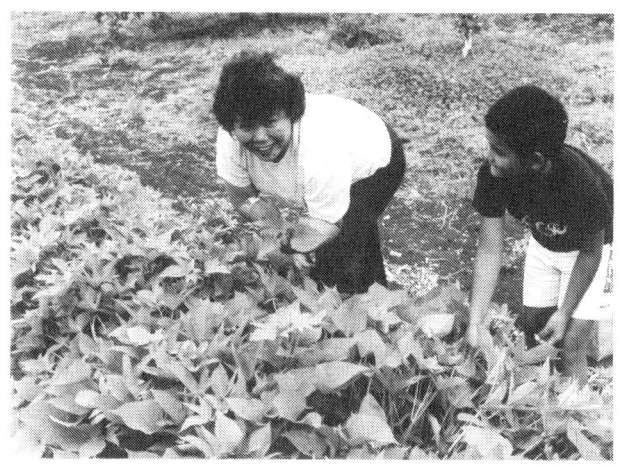

Midge Eli *(Coordinator, Wai'anae Diet)* **and Reagan O'Connor** *(son of Helen O'Connor, former Coordinator of the Moloka'i Diet and Wai'anae Diet Program)* **pick 'uala leaves in Wai'anae.**

The Wai'anae Diet Menu

Menu 1	**Menu 2**	**Menu 3**
(Breakfast)	*(Breakfast)*	*(Breakfast)*
taro/'ulu/'uala	taro/'ulu/'uala	taro/'ulu/'uala
fruit	fruit	fruit
Hawaiian tea	Hawaiian tea	Hawaiian tea
(Snack)	*(Snack)*	*(Snack)*
taro/'ulu/'uala	taro/'ulu/'uala	taro/'ulu/'uala
Hawaiian tea	Hawaiian tea	Hawaiian tea
(Lunch)	*(Lunch)*	*(Lunch)*
lawalu fish	grilled fish	steamed fish
poi	poi	poi
watercress salad	luau	cooked 'uala leaf
taro/'ulu/'uala	tomato salad	taro/'ulu/'uala
fruit	fruit	fruit
Hawaiian tea	Hawaiian tea	Hawaiian tea
(Snack)	*(Snack)*	*(Snack)*
taro/'ulu/'uala	taro/ulu/'uala	taro/'ulu/'uala
Hawaiian tea	Hawaiian tea	Hawaiian tea
(Dinner)	*(Dinner)*	*(Dinner)*
chicken luau	steamed fish	lawalu chicken
poi	poi	poi
watercress salad	luau leaf	'uala leaf salad
taro/'ulu/'uala	tomato salad	taro/'ulu/'uala
fruit	fruit	fruit
Hawaiian tea	Hawaiian tea	Hawaiian tea
(Snack)	*(Snack)*	*(Snack)*
taro/'ulu/'uala	taro/'ulu/'uala	taro/'ulu/'uala
Hawaiian tea	Hawaiian tea	Hawaiian tea

. . . limu to be offered as available.

. . . raw fish offered by individual request only.

Food and Recipes

PRINCIPAL FOODS

Kalo *(Taro)*

The old style of cooking kalo was by steaming in the imu *(underground covered cooking pit with hot rocks)*. However, kalo is usually prepared by boiling in a pot these days.

Boiled Kalo — Cut off the stem and lightly scrub the unpeeled kalo to remove dirt and roots. Place the larger kalo at the bottom of a pot and the smaller ones on top so they can be removed earlier as they cook. Add water to cover. Cover the pot and boil over medium heat until fork tender.

Note: Thoroughly cook kalo to avoid an itchy mouth.

Cool under cold water and then scrape off the skin with a dull knife or a spoon. Slice or cube kalo and serve warm or cold.

Steamed Kalo — Wash two medium-sized kalo and put into a medium-sized steamer with the water filled to one-half in the pot. Steam the kalo for one and a half hours or when fork tender. Cool under cold water and then scrape off the outer skin with a dull knife or a spoon. Slice or cube kalo and serve warm or cold.

KALO *(Taro)*

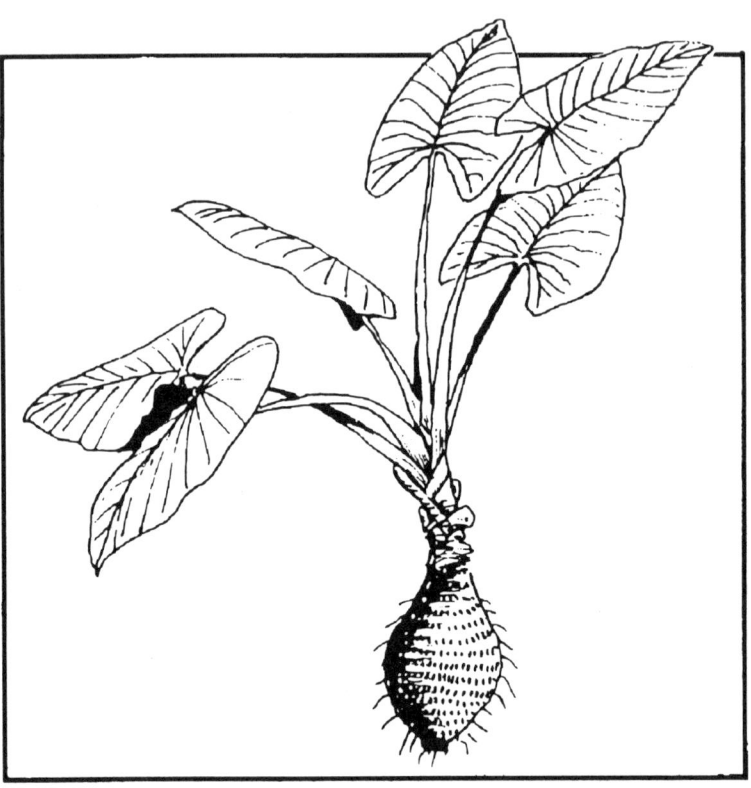

Kalo *(taro)* was the staff of life of the Hawaiian people. It has strong mana, and had much to do with sustaining the large population of human beings over hundreds of years.

Poi *(Kalo Poi)*

Poi was undoubtedly the most widely consumed food among the Native Hawaiians. Because kalo poi comes from kalo, it was believed to have the same powerful mana as did kalo. It was pounded from cooked kalo into a smooth texture. Poi is eaten as is, fresh or day old, or even a week old. In ancient Hawai'i, pa'i'ai poi could be preserved for many weeks if wrapped in ti and specially stored.

Poi is an excellent weight loss food, because an average 175-pound person would have to eat 9 pounds of poi to maintain his or her weight. *(Who can eat that much poi in a day, day after day?!)* Because poi is so low in calories, it can help you lose weight.

'ULU *(Breadfruit)*

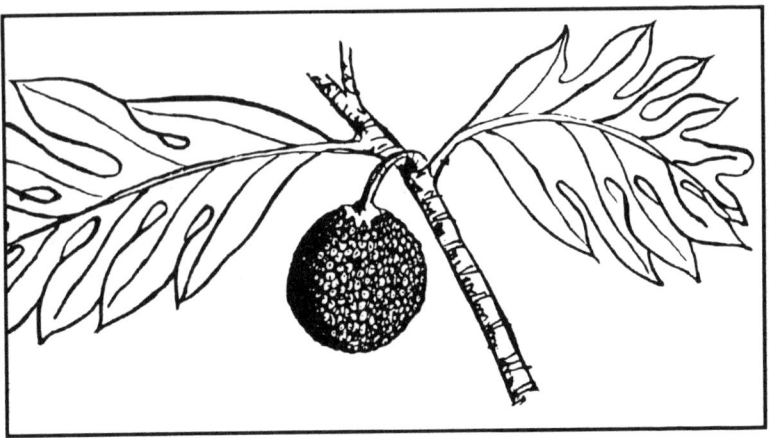

According to Hawaiian mythology, Ku saved his family during a famine when he planted himself into the ground and his head sprouted into a breadfruit tree.

'Ulu *(Breadfruit)*

Like kalo *(taro)*, 'ulu was another staple food in the Hawaiian diet. Nutritional value included starch, fiber, and B vitamins. Modes of preparation included baking, steaming, and pounding into poi.

Baked 'Ulu — Wash a ripe 'ulu and place in a pan with a small amount of water *(to keep the pan from burning)* in a preheated 400°F oven for one hour. Test to see if it is soft by poking it with a bamboo skewer. Twist the stem off, and core. Slice into bite-sized pieces.

Steamed 'Ulu — Remove the skin, stem and core. Slice into bite-sized pieces. Steam in a steamer for two hours, or cook in a pressure cooker for one hour.

'UALA *(Sweet Potato)*

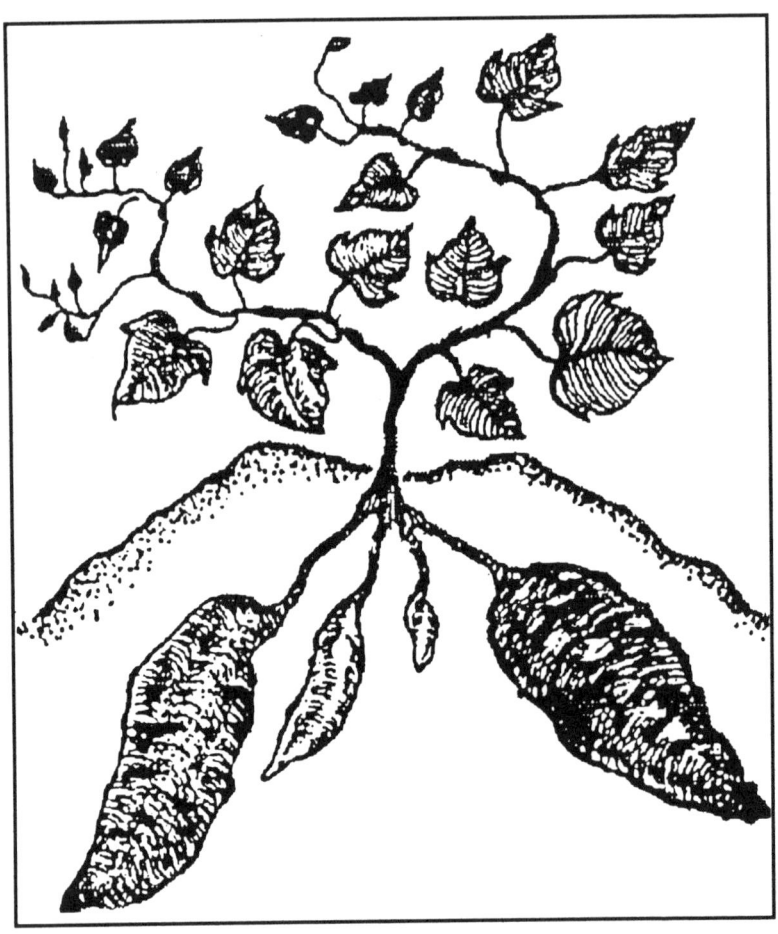

'Uala was considered to be an embodiment of Lono's "kinolau" animal form, Kamapua'a.

'Uala *(Sweet Potato)*

There were said to to be 230 varieties of sweet potato in ancient times, but today there are thought to be 24 varieties. Sweet potato was used as a staple in its whole form and in the form of poi. It was also used as a dessert mixed with coconut cream in the form of "paele 'uala." A brew was made from 'uala that was known as "'uala 'awa'awa."

Steamed 'Uala — Wash 'uala and pur about 3/4"-1" of water into a pot or steamer. Place the sweet potato on the steamer rack and steam for 25-30 minutes or until fork tender.

If you have a rice cooker, place enough water in the bottom to cover the first joint of your index finger and place the 'uala on the rack. Turn on the rice cooker and when it turns itself off the 'uala would be done.

UHI *(Yam)*

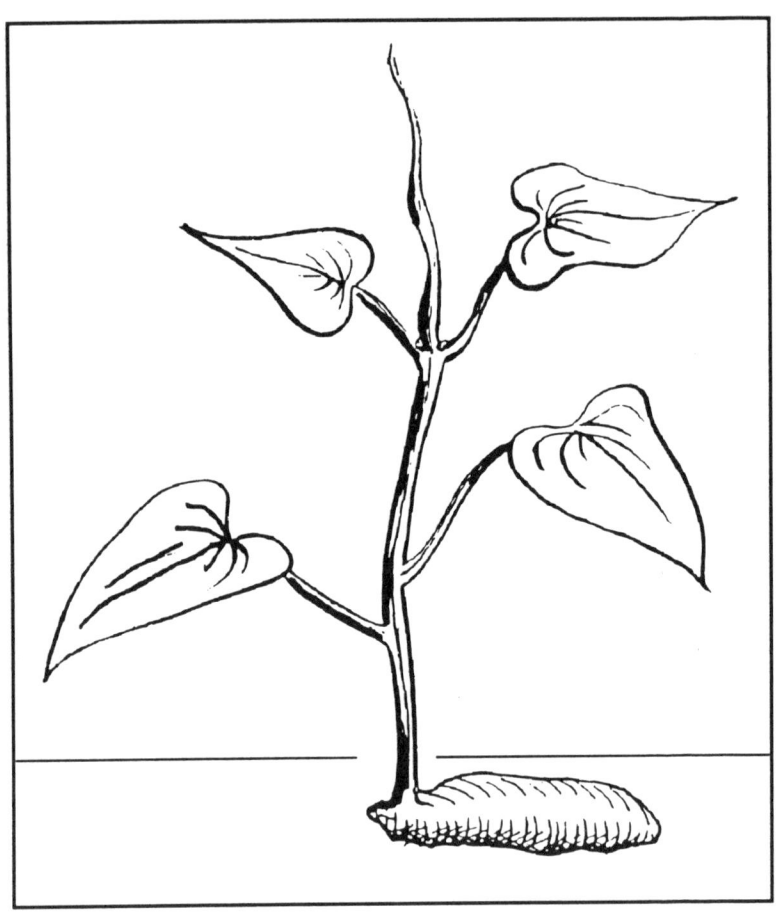

Uhi *(Yam)*

Uhi or yam, was not as important a staple in Hawai'i as in other areas of Polynesia. However, Captain Cook noted that it was grown in abundance on Ni'ihau, where it was difficult to grow kalo due to the dry climate. Nutritional value included starch, fiber, and vitamin A. It was prepared by steaming and baking, but was too mealy to be pounded into poi.

Steamed Uhi — Uhi or yams can be prepared in a similar manner as 'uala *(sweet potato)* but cooked for a shorter period of time of 20-25 minutes or until tender. *(See sweet potato cooking methods.)* For the rice cooker method, use a little less water.

Acceptable Principal Foods

See the Wai'anae Diet Transition Diet Program section for recipes.

- Brown rice
- Whole Wheat and Whole Wheat Products
- Potato
- Noodles
- Oatmeal
- Barley
- Corn
- Other Whole Grains

LUʻAU LEAF AND HAHA

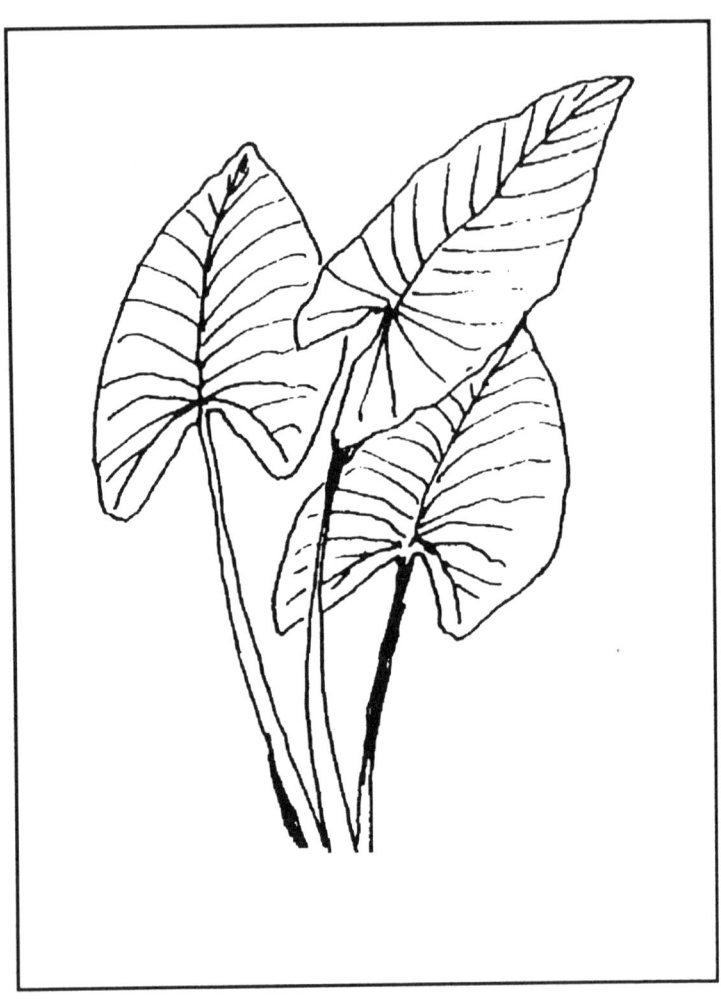

VEGETABLES

Lu'au Leaf

Lu'au leaf comes from the kalo plant. It is a delicious addition to any Hawaiian meal. It is high in vitamin A, calcium, iron and folic acid.

Lu'au leaf must be cooked because *(like the kalo)* it is itchy unless cooked properly. Cooking is simple, usually by boiling or steaming.

Preparation — Wash one pound of lu'au leaf and remove the haha *(stems)*. Put into a large pot with 1 quart of water and 3 pinches of Hawaiian salt. You may add diced onions for spice, if you like. Boil for 30 minutes.

Haha

Haha is the stem of the kalo plant. Like the lu'au leaf, it is delicious cooked by itself, or with other foods. It should NOT be eaten raw.

Preparation — Take the haha from the kalo leaf, wash, and strip the skin. Cut into roughly 1-inch pieces. Place in boiling water with a pinch of salt and simmer for 10 minutes.

'UALA LEAF (Sweet Potato Leaf)

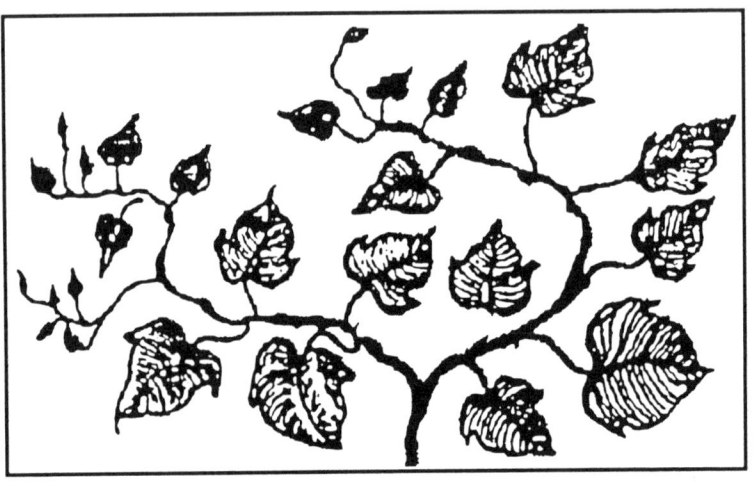

'Uala Leaf *(Sweet Potato Leaf)*

'Uala leaf is a delicious type of greens that was eaten as well. One trick in having delicious sweet potato greens is to pick the young tender shoots to eat. These will grow back in a short time, and you can have a regular supply if you grow 'uala in your yard.

Preparation — Take a large handful of young 'uala leaves and place into boiling water for approximately 5 minutes.

HOʻIʻO *(Fern)*

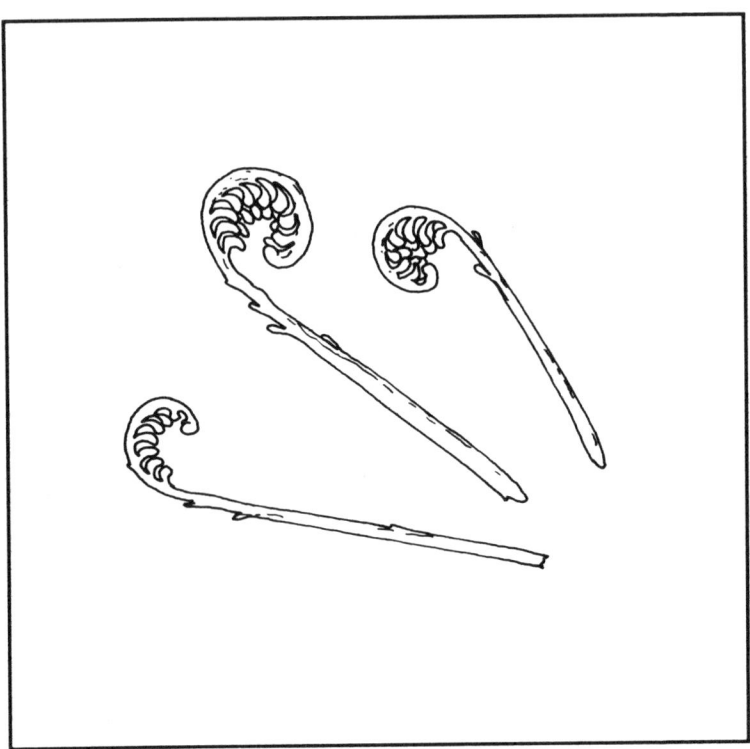

Ho'i'o *(Fern)*

Ho'i'o, or fern, was a delicacy in ancient times. It was found in the mountains, usually in moist areas. The young shoots were eaten as a side dish for variety. Today this fern can be found in the supermarkets as "warabi." Just ask your grocer or call Honolulu Poi Company, where it is sold.

Ho'i'o Salad — Soak 2 pounds of ho'i'o in water for a half hour. Rinse off and blanche in hot water. Cut into quarter-inch pieces and put into a large bowl. Mix in 7 medium, diced tomatoes and 5 medium, diced Maui onions. Chill before serving.

LIMU *(Seaweed)*

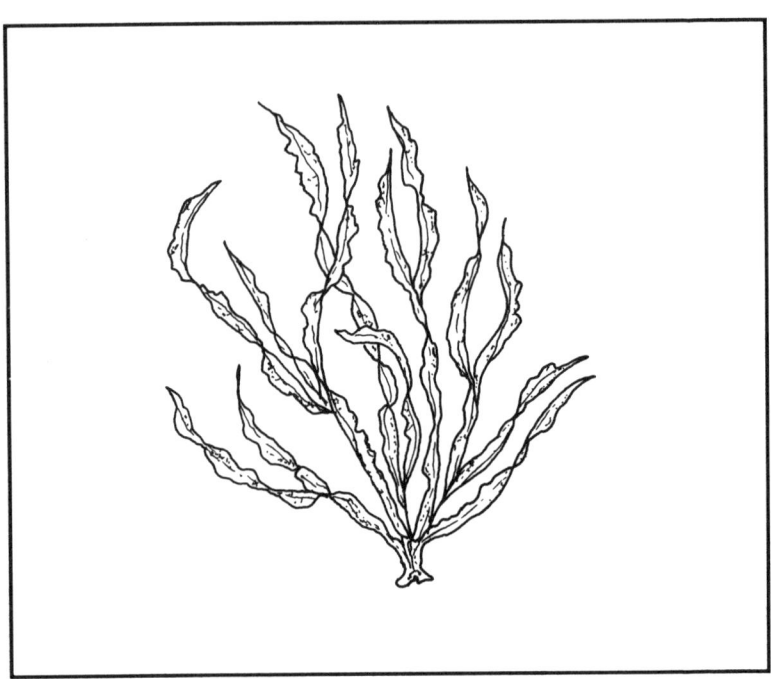

Limu *(Seaweed)*

Limu, or seaweed, was a regular side dish for the Hawaiians. It was naturally salty, and thus was used as a condiment to add to other foods. There were many, many varieties, most of which are no longer used.

Ele'ele *(black limu)* – fresh, brackish, or oceanside

Chop Chop

Lipoa – fragrant and tasty

Manauea *(ogo)* – fresh, salted vegetable, and poki

Kohu *(small, redish)* – an aliʻi limu

Wawaeʻiole "rats feet" *(miru)*; pokpoklo *(Filipino)* – very common. Prepared with sea urchin *(ʻakiʻaki)* – very tough.

Other Greens

Popolo Leaf and **ʻAweoweo** *(Lambs' Quarters)*.

Many other greens were also used but may be unavailable today.

Acceptable Vegetable Substitutes

See the Waiʻanae Diet Transition Diet Program section for recipes.

- Broccoli
- Spinach
- Kale
- Collard Greens
- Califlower
- Squash
- Peas
- Lettuce
- Watercress
- Carrots
- Corn
- Pumpkin
- Onions
- String beans
- Celery
- Cabbage
- Bok Choy
- Other Vegetables

MAIʻA *(Banana)*

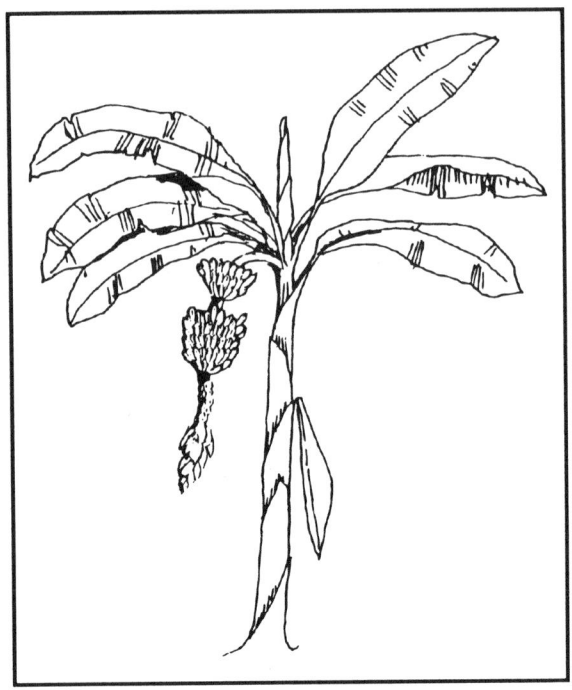

Maiʻa was one of the fruits brought over by the original Hawaiians.

ʻOHIʻA ʻAI *(Mountain Apple)*

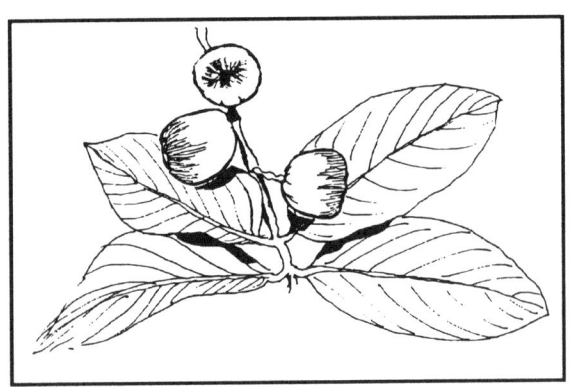

FRUITS

Fruit *(Hua)*

Fruit was a natural dessert for the ancient Hawaiians. The most common fruits were Mai'a *(Banana)* and 'Ohi'a'ai *(Mountain Apple)*. Today, almost all fruits are acceptable substitutes and provide a delicious variety for regular use.

Mai'a *(Banana)*

Baked Bananas — You should use ripe cooking bananas *(outside should have brown spots and no green coloration)*. Place unpeeled bananas in a steaming basket, or pot with a little water to cover bottom. Steam 5 to 12 minutes until skins split.

Microwave Bananas — Place in a dish with 2 or 3 tablespoons of water. Microwave 2 to 4 minutes until skin splits. Peel, slice and serve hot on a platter.

Acceptable Fruit Substitutes

See the Wai'anae Diet Transition Diet Program section for recipes.

- Apples
- Oranges
- Lemons
- Pears
- Papaya
- Pineapple
- Peaches
- Strawberries
- Nectarines
- Guava
- Mango
- Other Fruits

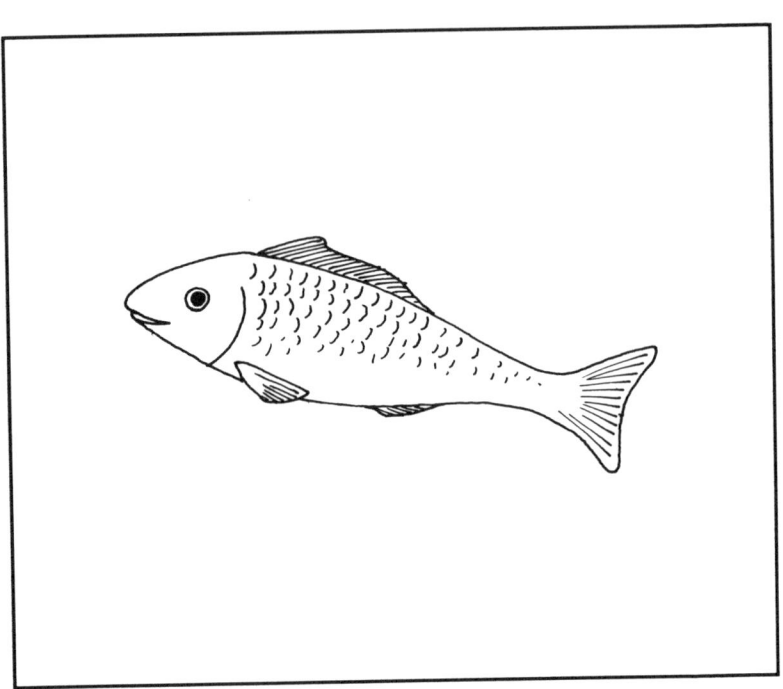

PROTEIN FOODS

Fish *(I'a)*

As with all island people, fish was an important source of food. However, it was not the "main dish," but rather another side dish. The main dish was the kalo or the poi. Some meals consisted simply of kalo, fruit and greens. Fish was not eaten at every meal. The reason we know fish or any fowl or animal food was not eaten at every meal is because there were no refrigerators then. When fish was eaten, it was cooked simply over a fire *(pulehu)* and seasoned with a pinch of salt at the table, or steamed in the imu or as in lawalu style.

Mullet was a prized fish and can be eaten raw or cooked.

Other favorites are:

Uhu	'O'opu
'Opelu	'Opae
Manini	'Opihi
Kumu	Other Seafood

Lawalu

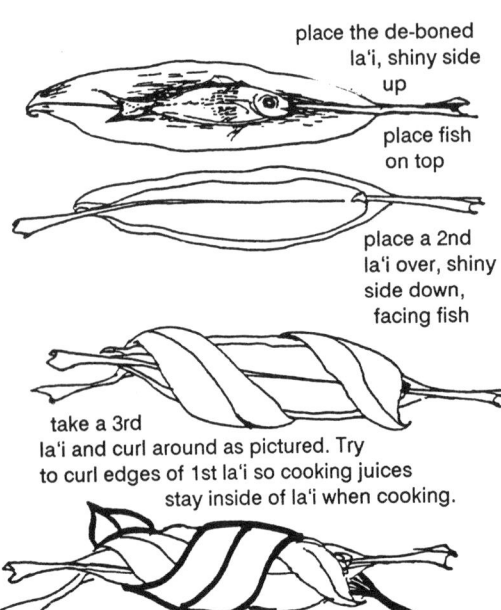

place the de-boned la'i, shiny side up

place fish on top

place a 2nd la'i over, shiny side down, facing fish

take a 3rd la'i and curl around as pictured. Try to curl edges of 1st la'i so cooking juices stay inside of la'i when cooking.

take a 4th la'i and curl around as pictured

Lawalu

Lawalu is a fish, or meat, or dough, bound in la'i and broiled on coals or ashes.

Some fish were favored for lawalu, especially 'o'opu: kumu and weke were also used.

take the loose ends of stems and tie each end

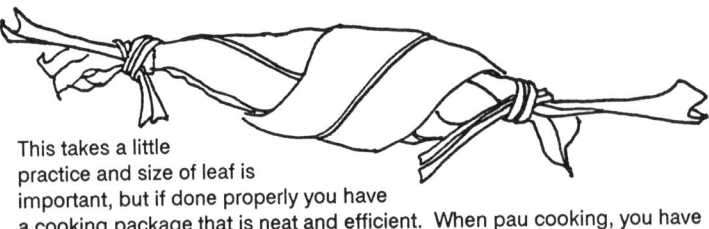

This takes a little practice and size of leaf is important, but if done properly you have a cooking package that is neat and efficient. When pau cooking, you have a nice la'i platter to eat from.

(drawings and text by Eric Enos from "Hawaiian Style" published by The 'Opelu Project Inc., Wai'anae, HI)

Lawalu

Baked Lawalu Fish or Chicken —

- 1-1/2 lbs. fresh fish fillets
  or
- 2-1/2 lbs. whole fish *(i.e., Kumu, Mullet, Moana or Moi)*
  or
- 2-1/2 lbs. chicken
- rock salt
- several ti *(laʻi)* leaves
- luau leaves

Scale and clean fish and rub with rock salt. Wrap the fish or chicken in several luʻau leaves, then in ti leaves *(laʻi)*, and secure ends with string. Bake at 350°F for 1 to 1-1/2 hours for whole fish *(depending on size)*, 30 to 35 minutes for fillets, and 2 hours for chicken. For the fish, if desired, add bay leaves and sliced round or green onion on each fish or fillet before wrapping. Salt to taste and serve.

Steamed Lawalu Fish or Chicken — one serving

- 5-7 taro leaves
- 3 ounces of chicken or deboned fish
- 2 ti *(laʻi)* leaves
- pinch of sea salt *(optional)*

Cut taro stems off from the taro leaf. Wash taro leaves. Stack 5 to 7 taro leaves on each other. Place the chicken or fish in the center of the taro leaves. Add a pinch of salt. Follow the instructions on page 68 and wrap the taro leaves to cover the chicken or fish. Wrap the taro leaves and chicken or fish in ti leaves as shown and steam in a covered container for 4 hours.

Chicken *(Moa)*

Along with pigs, chickens were brought over the seas with the original kanaka maoli. Chicken was eaten even less frequently in ancient times than fish. It can be prepared in a similar fashion to fish, as in lawalu style, or pulehu style. Today, we know it is better to remove the skin of the chicken because of the high fat content.

Chicken Haha —

- 2 pounds of haha *(stems of taro leaf)*
- 5 pounds of chicken *(deboned, skinned or cubed)*
- 1 medium diced Maui onion
- 1 medium shredded garlic clove.

In 2 cups of boiling water, simmer the haha for 15 to 20 minutes. Brown the chicken with onions and garlic. Add the haha and simmer for 30 minutes. Serve hot.

Acceptable Protein Food Substitutes

See the Waiʻanae Diet Transition Diet Program section for recipes.

- Tofu
- Beans
- Lentils
- Turkey
- Shrimp
- Other low-fat protein foods

THE WAI'ANAE DIET TRANSITION DIET PROGRAM

The Wai'anae Diet "Transition Diet" is part of the Wai'anae Diet Program. A common misconception is that the Wai'anae Diet Program is a diet exclusively of traditional Hawaiian food. This misconception often leads to the question about "How do we expect people to stay on the diet when Hawaiian foods are so expensive?"

Actually, the Wai'anae Diet Program used the traditional Hawaiian diet as a model and encourages the use of traditional foods from other cultures. The enables people to make a "transition" into everyday life with inexpensive foods such as brown rice, broccoli and other familiar staples and vegetables.

Meanwhile, we encourage the use of and the interest in growing taro, poi, and other traditional Hawaiian foods. We hope that by our efforts we can help enhance the value of these foods or that these industries may thrive, ultimately, we hope that this will contribute to increasing the supply and decreasing the cost of these foods. Until that happens we hope you enjoy maintaining your health with the Wai'anae Diet transition diet foods.

The Wai'anae Transition Diet Menu

Menu 1

(Breakfast)
oatmeal w/raisins
fruit
non-caloric beverage
i.e., grain coffee

(Snack)
sweet potato

(Lunch)
corn on the cob
vegetable soup
fruit

(Dinner)
savory garbanzo beans
steamed/baked squash
watercress salad
steamed kale
fruit
herb tea

Menu 2

(Breakfast)
fruit
whole wheat toast
no-sugar fruit preserves
non-caloric beverage

(Snack)
fruit

(Lunch)
grilled fish
brown rice
squash
vegetables

(Dinner)
spaghetti
greens/salad
cooked greens
whole wheat bread
fruit
herb tea

Menu 3

(Breakfast)
oatmeal w/raisins
skim milk
fruit
herb tea

(Snack)
sweet potato

(Lunch)
baked potato
steamed vegetables
salad
fruit

(Dinner)
baked fish
brown rice
salad
cooked vegetable
fruit
herb tea

Transition Recipes

PRINCIPAL FOODS

Long-Grain Brown Rice

If at all possible, you should learn to use a stainless steel pressure cooker for brown rice. It tastes much better and cooks much more quickly *(see instructions below)*. If not you can use a regular pot or a rice cooker as follows.

Steam-cooked Rice — Cook enough so that you can have some for tomorrow's lunch.

- 2 cups long-grain brown rice
- 4 cups of water
- 1 pinch sea salt

Gently wash rice until the water rinses clear. If you have time, soak for 2 to 6 hours. Place in a 2-quart pot *(stainless steel if possible)*. Pour water to cover the rice. Add sea salt. Cover, bring to a boil, reduce flame, simmer for 45 minutes to one hour. Remove from flame. Let sit for 10 minutes before serving. *(Do not uncover rice while cooking.)* Makes 6 cups of cooked rice.

Rice-Cooker Rice — If you use an automatic rice cooker, use two cups of water to each cup of rice. Wash and rinse the rice, add the water and turn on the cooker. Adjust the water to your liking.

Pressure-cooked Rice — For Pressure Cooked Brown Rice use 3-1/2 cups of water. Wash rice and soak 2 to 6 hours *(it will take a little longer to cook if not pre-soaked)*. Place rice and water into a pressure cooker *(stainless steel if possible)*. Add salt, cover lid as directed by manufacturer of pressure cooker. Bring to pressure on high heat then lower to low heat and cook for 35 to 45 minutes. Let pressure come down, then let stand for 5 to 10 minutes, stir and serve.

For Breakfast – Brown Rice and Quick Miso Soup —

Try to learn to use real miso if it is available because it is easy to use and is better than a dry mix.

- wakame flakes
- Shiitake mushrooms, 4 pieces crumbled *(optional)*
- 4 cups water
- miso

Boil water. Measure 2 tablespoons of miso *(or to taste)* into a cup and add a small amount of the water to make a puree of the miso. Add the puree back to the soup and add wakame flakes and crumbled shiitake mushroom peices. Simmer for about 2 minutes. Garnish with scallions or add other vegetables as desired.

Instant Miso Soup — If you must use an instant miso soup mix, add mushrooms, wakame flakes and other vegetables if you wish.

Spaghetti and Tomato Sauce —

- 1 pkg spaghetti noodles *(preferrably whole wheat or spinach type)*
- 1 bottle prepared spaghetti sauce
- 1 cup fresh or canned mushrooms

Cook whole grain spaghetti according to directions on package. Drain and toss lightly. You may add dried parsley. Serve with no oil or low oil tomato sauce from the health food store and tossed greens with no-oil dressing.

Baked Rice and Shiitake Mushrooms —

- 2 cups brown rice
- 4 to 5 shiitake mushrooms *(fresh or dried)*
- pinch sea salt per cup of grain
- low sodium soy sauce
- water

Rinse brown rice until water rinses clear. Soak mushrooms in 1/4 to 1/2 cup of water until soft. Reserve soak water. Slice mushrooms into thin slices. In oblong baking dish, place the rinsed, drained brown rice, the shiitake mushrooms, sea salt, and about two tablespoons of low sodium soy sauce. Mix together so that the mushrooms are evenly distributed throughout the rice. Add three 1/2 cups of water. Cover baking dish and bake in 350° oven for 45 to 60 minutes. Remove from oven and allow to sit for 10 to 15 minutes, remove cover and serve. Serve with tossed greens with no-oil dressing.

Corn on the Cob — Peel the husks off the ears of corn. Remove any bad spots. Place about 1-1/2 inches of water in bottom of a pan. Bring to boil, cover, and reduce flame to low setting. Cook for 3 to 5 minutes and turn ears a time or two to ensure even cooking. Remove from pan and serve to a platter.

You can eat it plain *(Hawaii has delicious sweet corn)* or, ume paste makes a nice condiment to use on the corn instead of the usual butter or margarine. Just spread a little umeboshi paste on the corn and this makes the corn taste even sweeter. Umeboshi vinegar is also very tasty. Just remember that these condiments are high in salt.

VEGETABLES

Steamed Cabbage —

- 1/2 head cabbage, shredded
- pinch sea salt

Place the cabbage and sea salt in a pan. Add enough water to steam. Cover and bring to a boil. Reduce the flame and simmer for 5 to 7 minutes or just until tender but still bright green. The sea salt will bring out the sweetness. Remove to a serving dish. Serve with Garlic Bread.

Steamed Collard Greens —

- 2 large bunches collard greens
- water

Wash the collard leaves thoroughly, and slice on the diagonal into bite-sized pieces. Place in 1-1/2 inches of water and cover pan and bring to a boil. Reduce flame and steam for 5 to 10 minutes or just until tender but still bright green. Remove from flame right away and serve to retain bright green color.

Steamed Kale Greens —

- 1 or 2 large bunches of kale greens
- water

Wash kale leaves thoroughly and cut on the diagonal into bite-size pieces. Place about 1-1/2 cups water in pan, add the chopped greens, cover and bring to a boil. Reduce the flame and steam greens until just tender but still bright green. Remove to a serving dish right away to retain bright green color. Serve with tofu dressing.

Tofu Dressing for Steamed Vegetables

- 1/2 block of tofu *(medium firm is preferable)*
- 1 clove garlic, minced
- 1 tablespoon tahini or 1 tablespoon seasame oil
- 1 teaspoon miso
- 1 tablespoon lemon juice
- *(optional)* other ingredients of your choice such as parsley, mustard, curry powder, umeboshi plum

Blend all ingredients until creamy smooth. Be careful. Tofu spoils easily, so if you want to keep it an extra day, steam it for 3 minutes before blending and refrigerate dressing immediately while not in use.

Steamed Kabocha Squash *(acorn squash may be used)* —

Scrub the squash really clean, cut in half, remove the seeds, then slice into quarters. Place in pot *(in a steamer basket, if desired)* in which 1-1/2 inches of water has been placed. Cover and slowly cook for about 20 to 30 minutes or until it tests tender with a toothpick. Remove to a serving dish.

Steamed Greens and Summer Squash —

- 2 big bunches kale greens, wash and chop
- 2 to 3 medium-sized summer squash
- pinch of sea salt
- water

Pour about 1-1/2 inches of water into a pan, add a pinch of sea salt, then the greens, then the squash. Cover the pan and bring to a boil. Reduce flame to a medium heat and cook 5 to 8 minutes or until the greens are just bright green and tender. Remove from the pan, drain and serve.

Baked Buttercup Squash —

- 1 medium large buttercup squash
- pinch of sea salt
- 1/2 cup water

Scrub squash, cut in half and remove seeds, then cut into quarters. Add water to baking dish, add sea salt, place squash in baking dish, cover and bake in 350° oven for 45 minutes or until squash tests tender when pierced with a toothpick. Place in serving dish and serve.

Wakame with Carrots *(or other vegetables)* —

- 1/2 ounces dried wakame
- 2 cups large chunks of carrots
  (or other vegetables such as cauliflower, turnips, daikon, celery burdock or lotus root)
- water
- 2 to 3 teaspoons low-sodium soy sauce
- scallions or parsley sprigs for garnish *(optional)*

Rinse and soak wakame. Slice into into large pieces. Put the carrots *(or other vegetables)* in a pot, and add water to half cover the carrots. Bring to a boil, cover and reduce the heat to low. Simmer until the carrots are nearly done *(about 20 to 30 minutes. Adjust cooking time for othe vegetables)*. Then add the wakame and low-sodium soy sauce to taste and simmer until carrots are done. Garnish.

Hijiki with Onions *(or other vegetables)* —

- 1/2 ounce dried hijiki (or arame)
- 1/4 teaspoon dark sesame oil
- 1 onion *(or other vegetables such as carrots, burdock root, lotus root, or tofu)*
- water
- 1 to 2 tablespoon low-sodium soy sauce

Wash and drain the hijiki. After washing, be sure to place in a separate bowl to eliminate any sand that may be present. Then soak hijiki for about 10 minutes. While soaking, slice onion vertically into thin crescents. Lighly oil a frying pan heat it. Add the onions and a little water and saute for 2 to 3 minutes. Place the hijiki on top of the onions and add water to cover the onions. Bring to a boil, turn the heat to low, and add a small amount of low-sodium soy sauce. Cover and simmer for about 40 minutes (depending on the vegetable. Add soy sauce to taste. Simmer for another 15 minutes, or until the liquid is almost gone.

Wakame is a leafy Japanese seaweed that is an excellent substitute for Hawaiian limu. It is found in the Japanese section of the supermarket or at most health food stores. As in other seaweeds, it is high in calcium.

An easy way to use wakame is to crumble or cut it into small pieces while dry or use wakame flakes *(also known as "fueru wakame")* and sprinkle some in any soup.

Hijiki is a stringy seaweed also found in the Japanese section of the supermarket or at health food stores. It initially has a strong ocean smell that is easily cooked off. It is the highest in calcium of commonly eaten seaweed.

FRUITS

Cantaloupe Strawberry "Gelatin" —

- 1 cantaloupe
- 3 small boxes strawberries
- 6 cups water
- 2 cups apple juice
- 5 bars agar

Make cantaloupe into balls and reserve juice to add to mixture. Add water to juice. Break agar into this mixture, soak until dissolved. Bring to a boil, reduce flame, and simmer for 20 to 30 minutes. Partially chill, add cantaloupe balls and strawberries. Refrigerate and chill until completely firm.

Baked Apples —

- 1 large apple for each person
  (*try Rome or Granny Smith*)
- Sunflower seeds, roasted
- Raisins
- 1/4 to 1/2 teaspoon vanilla
- 1/4 to 1/2 teaspoon cinnamon

Wash apples well. Slice off and save the tops of the apples. Core the apples about 1 inches down into the apple, being careful not to poke through the bottom. Mix all the other ingredients and fill the apples. Replace the top slice of the apple, and bake at 375° for 30 to 45 minutes until tender. For juicer apples, cover halfway through cooking. Add 1/4 cup water to bottom of pan for moisture.

Cinnamon Applesauce —

- 4 apples
- 1/4 cup raisins
- 3/4 teaspoon cinnamon
- 1 cup water
- 1 cup apple juice
- 1 heaping tablespoon arrowroot or cornstarch

Peel and slice the apples. Mix raisins, cinnamon and water in a saucepan. Place apple slices in mixture. Bring to a boil, cover, and simmer for 10 to 15 minutes, or until apples are tender. Dissolve the arrowroot or cornstarch in cold apple juice, add and stir until thick.

PROTEIN FOODS

Savory Garbanzo Beans —

- 1 cup garbanzo beans
- 1 strip konbu
- 1 tablespoon miso
- 1/2 onion chopped
- 1 clove garlic crushed *(optional)*

Wash garbanzo beans and soak in water 6 to 12 hours. You can soak it in the morning for an evening meal, for example. Soak Konbu in water just before cooking for a few minutes until soft. Rinse off konbu and cut into 1-inch long strips. Place beans and konbu in a pressure cooker or pot. Add water to cover beans well. Dilute miso in the water. Pressure cook for 35 to 40 minutes or boil in a pot for 3 to 4 hours *(in either case, bring to boil on high then turn to low heat)*.

Black Bean With Onion —

- 2 cups black beans
- 5 cups water
- 1 medium onion, diced
- 1 teaspoon sea salt
- 1 teaspoon cumin seeds

Sort through beans for stones. Wash beans and soak for 4 to 6 hours before cooking. Pressure cook for 45 minutes or bring to a boil, covered, and reduce flame to low and simmer for 1 to 2 hours. Add sea salt 30 to 45 minutes before serving. Adding salt to beans at the beginning of cooking time prevents beans from becoming tender. Add cumin near end of cooking. Good also served chilled as a side dish or when added to salad.

Transition recipes provided by Terry Shintani, M.D.

RESULTS OF THE WAI'ANAE DIET

New Study Shows Ancient Hawaiian Diet Cures Modern Ills — Hawaiian Diet Also Causes Automatic Weight Loss

Reversal of serious illness and weight loss without limiting calories was demonstrated by a non-calorie restricted traditional Hawaiian diet at the Waianae Coast Comprehensive Health Center in Hawaii. An average weight loss of 17.1 pounds per person was noted along with reversal of heart disease, high blood pressure, and diabetes in a study involving 19 Native Hawaiian adults over a period of just three weeks. This was even more remarkable because Hawaiians have among the highest rates of obesity and death from these diseases in the nation. The results of this study were published in the world's leading nutrition journal, the American Journal of Clinical Nutrition, by Terry Shintani, M.D., M.P.H., Hawaiian nutritionist Claire Hughes, M.S., R.D., Helen Kanawaliwali O'Connor, C.H.W., and Sheila Beckham, M.P.H., R.D.C. in the June 1991 edition.

In this program, known as the Wai'anae Diet Program (WDP), Native Hawaiians were placed on a diet consisting of exclusively Native Hawaiian foods *(available before Western contact)* for a period of 21 days. They were allowed to eat as much as they wanted with the exception of some restriction on the quantity of animal protein. Results indicated an average weight loss of 17.1 pounds over 21 days. In addition, cholesterol fell 14.1% from an average of 222.3 mg/dl to an average of 191 mg/dl, with a slight improvement in HDL to cholesterol ration. Triglycerides, a risk factor for heart disease improved as well, falling from an average of 211.3 to 163 mg/dl. Blood sugar control improved in all seven individuals with diabetes on the program with the overall blood sugar level decreasing from 161.9 to 123.4 mg/dl. One individual who was on 60 units of insulin per day no longer needs any diabetes medication one year later. There was no increase in exercise on the program and analysis of the intake revealed that participants ate more food on the diet but ingested fewer calories.

The WDP was designed in response to the tragic irony that in Hawaii, the healthiest state in the union, Native Hawaiians have the shortest life-span as compared to all other ethnic groups in America. Most of the deaths are diet and obesity related. Hawaiians have among the highest rates of obesity in the nation with a prevalence of approximately 65%. By sharp contrast, early writings, photographs and drawings indicate that Hawaiians were of a "thin rather than full habit" (Stewart 1883). Diet-related diseases such as heart disease, stroke, cancer and diabetes were also rare in ancient Hawaiians.

The researchers believed that a change in the diet to modern foods rather than "overeating" is the cause of obesity and the deadly profile of modern diseases in Native Hawaiians today. In contrast to the high fat, high cholesterol modern diet, the Hawaiian diet was approximately 7 to 12% fat and high in complex carbohydrates and bulk. The principal foods on the diet was taro *(a starchy tuber)*, poi *(a mashed form of taro)*, sweet potatoes, yams, breadfruit, assorted greens, seaweed, fruit, small amounts of fish and occasionally chicken. Degree of satisfaction was measured, and it was determined to be relatively high during the program. The program also taught the subsitution of modern equivalent foods and modern recipes for maintenance of the healthy changes in the diet. This facilitates the use of the program concepts by the general public.

In addition, the WDP included Hawaiian healers to teach spiritual, mental, emotional as well as physical health as an integral part of the program. This is consistent with ancient Hawaiian cultural values. Community networking was also an integral part of the program and each participant was encouraged to be a teacher and promoter of the WDP's healthy lifestyle message. This approach is already yielding benefits as one participant has already caused 70 others to experience the program through their own collective efforts.

*Reprinted by permission of the Star Bulletin.

Weight loss a 'bonus'

By Linda Hosek
Star-Bulletin

A few years ago Ed Aikala weighed 425 pounds and spent up to $500 a month on medicine.

When he looked at a beautiful tree, he would think about being buried under it.

He even gave himself the last rites in a hospital when he couldn't get a breath of air. He heard the staff say: "We almost lost him."

Now the 6-foot-4 Aikala is down to 275 pounds, walks several miles a day and takes medication only for asthma.

Gone are the prescriptions for high blood pressure, insulin and diuretics, which combined made him feel like a zombie.

But he keeps empty pill containers in a garbage sack in his bathroom to remind him that he could die if he doesn't watch what he eats.

Aikala, a 50-year-old pure Hawaiian, credits his newfound health to a regime that was basic to his slender ancestors: the traditional Hawaiian diet.

He was one of 19 obese native Hawaiian adults who participated in a 21-day experiment to show that the traditional diet high in poi and sweet potatoes promotes health. The average weight of the participants was 246 pounds.

The study, known as the Waianae Diet Program, was published this month in the American Journal of Clinical Nutrition, a nutrition publication highly regarded worldwide.

Participants lost an average of 17.1 pounds, lowered their cholesterol by 14 percent and decreased their risk for heart disease, said Dr. Terry Shintani, who designed the study for the Waianae Coast Comprehensive Health Center.

"The weight loss was a bonus," Aikala said. "I'm just glad to be rid of all those medications."

Shintani said he initiated the study in response to a tragic irony: Native Hawaiians live in the country's healthiest state, but have the shortest life-span among the country's ethnic groups.

Pure Hawaiians are three times as likely to die of heart disease as the general U.S. population and twice as likely to die of cancer or a stroke. And they are six times as likely to die of diabetes.

Poor diet and obesity, which affects up to 65 percent of the native population of 200,000, cause most of the deaths, he said.

But their excess weight comes from modern eating habits, not overeating.

Many obese native Hawaiians consume high-fat, high-cholesterol foods, including plate lunches, fast food and canned food. The native diet is low-fat and high in complex carbohydrates and bulk.

Many obese native Hawaiians consume high-fat, high-cholesterol foods, including plate lunches, fast food and canned food. The native diet is low-fat and high in complex carbohydrates and bulk.

Although participants ate as much as they wanted of the traditional foods to avoid hunger, they consumed fewer calories and considerably less fat. Before the program, they ate an average of 2,594 calories, of which at least 40 percent was from fat, he said.

On the program, their caloric intake dropped to an average of 1,569, of which only about 7 percent was from fat. A regular diet should contain 10 to 20 percent fat, Shintani said.

Terry Shintani

"This demonstration project was to show that this is a healthful diet," Shintani said.

But he also hopes it will enable native Hawaiians to regain their self-esteem and socioeconomic stature in the community.

Hawaiians had been primarily taro farmers and fishermen in previous centuries. But the overthrow of the monarchy in 1897 changed their lifestyle and self-image.

"This loss of control over their own affairs hastened the downward spiral of the Hawaiians' economic, social and cultural condition," he said.

Many Hawaiians became sedentary and poor, suffering from stress. The Westernization of their diet contributed to their decline as many reached for fast foods instead of steaming sweet potatoes.

"I'm basically trying to change the secular trend — what Hawaiians do as a whole," Shintani said. "We picked people for the study to

# of healthful traditional diet

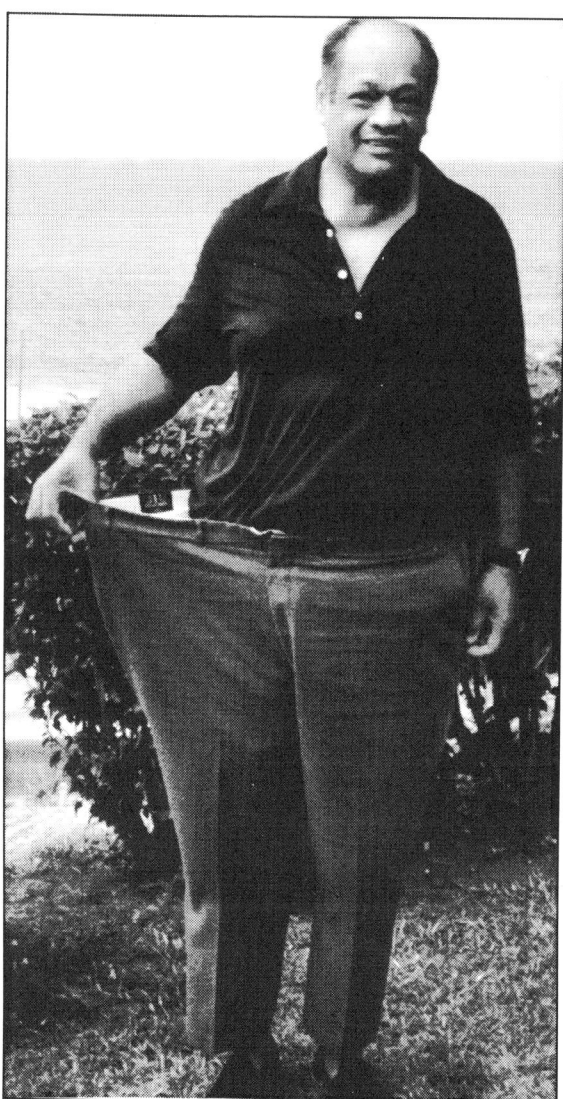

Special to the Star-Bulletin

Eddie Aikala has lost 150 pounds in the last few years by adopting the diet of his ancestors. He was one of 19 Hawaiians who participated in an experiment to show that the traditional diet promotes health.

seed the community."

He said he hoped to influence all Hawaiians, achieving at least a 10 percent drop in the amount of dietary fat Hawaiians consume in the next decade.

The general public also has begun to consume less dietary fat, dropping from about about 40 percent to 38 percent in recent years.

Shintani provided a broader, transition diet to enable the participants to stay on track. Additions include brown rice, potatoes, vegetables, beans, tofu, chicken, shrimp and turkey.

But staying on the diet can be tough "if the rest of the family eats what they want," said Hooipo DeCambra, a program participant.

"If people replace even one meal with brown rice or poi, they'll be in better shape," Shintani said.

DeCambra was so dedicated to the original program that she took her taro, sweet potatoes and luau to a dinner hosted by Barbara Bush in Washington, D.C. The dinner was part of a women's leadership summit on mammography.

"I could talk about the diet," said DeCambra, also an investigator for a breast-cancer screening project. "I told them we were trying to save ourselves."

The Waianae Diet Program was conducted without state or federal money.

"We asked everyone, but we got not a penny," Shintani said. "This was funded out of the blood and guts of the Hawaiian community."

Shintani said mainland researchers have received money to study Hawaiian health, but Hawaiians have received no benefits from the efforts.

"They end up saying we have health problems and disappear," he said.

Local contributions came from the Kahumana Community and the Honolulu Poi Co., which donated 400 pounds of poi, he said.

Shintani has received $38,000 from the Robert E. Black Foundation of the Hawaii Community Foundation for a second study to begin in September to measure the diet's long-term effects.

The original Waianae Diet Program also included spiritual, mental and emotional components. Participants had access to Hawaiian healers and learned control techniques, including positive imagery, breathing and meditation, Shintani said.

"Your whole body changes," DeCambra said. "Your personality is more pleasant, you have more energy and you appreciate your whole being so you take care of it."

DeCambra, who had to break her fast-food habit, is now an advocate of the traditional diet. But she and Shintani single out Aikala as the program's hero.

Now, instead of seeing a tree as shade for his grave, he sees himself watering it.

"I didn't think I could be this healthy," said Aikala, who had hospital bills exceeding $250,000. "The Hawaiians had something with their diet."

The health center has no funding for an ongoing traditional diet program, but it has produced "The Waianae Book of Hawaiian Health." Copies are available at $10 each. Write: Waianae Coast Comprehensive Health Center, 86-260 Farrington Highway, Waianae 96792.

91

Mortality Among Pure Hawaiians
As Compared to the Average Mortality Rates for All Races in the U.S.

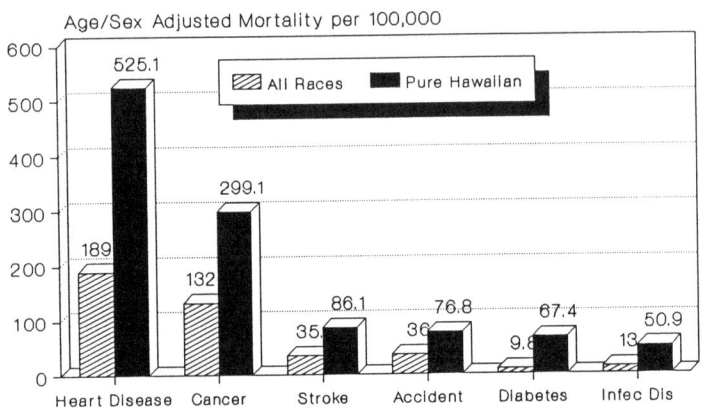

Source: Office of Technology Assessment
U.S. Congress, April, 1987

Mortality Among Native Hawaiians
As Compared to the Average Mortality Rates for All Races in the U.S.

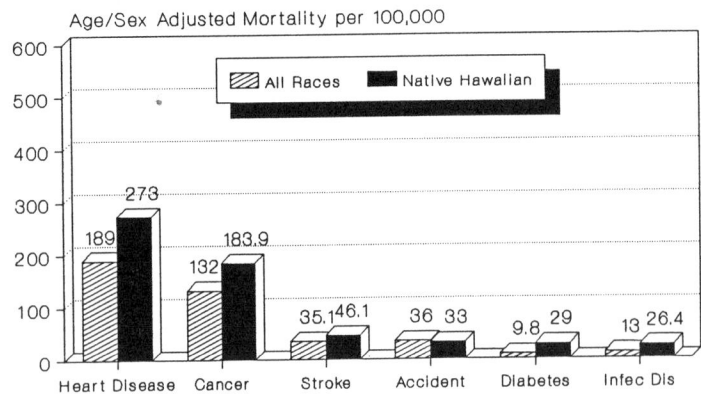

Source: Office of Technology Assessment
U.S. Congress, April, 1987

1. Mortality

The Wai'anae Diet Program was designed in response to the high rates of mortality among Native Hawaiians. Currently, 4 of the 6 leading causes of death among pure and part-Hawaiians are diet-related including heart disease, cancer, stroke and diabetes. These diet-related diseases account for approximately 70% of the deaths among Native Hawaiians.

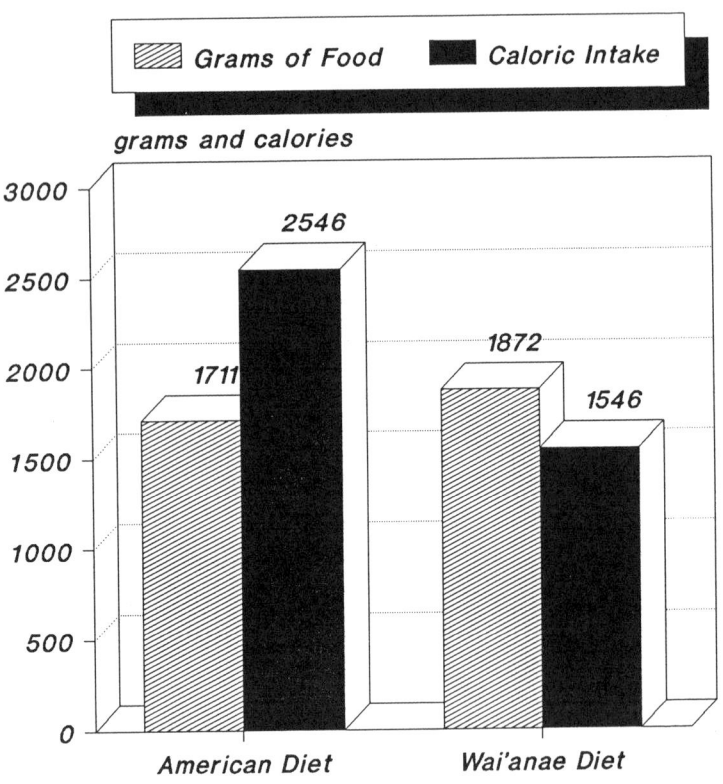

2. Weight Loss Without Counting Calories

Wai'anae Diet Program demonstrated that people could lose weight without counting calories. Participants ate until they were satisfied. They actually ate more food on the program than they did ordinarily. They ate 4.1 pounds of food a day compared to 3.7 pounds before the program. But they ate nearly 1,000 calories less and lost an average of 17 pounds per person in only three weeks.

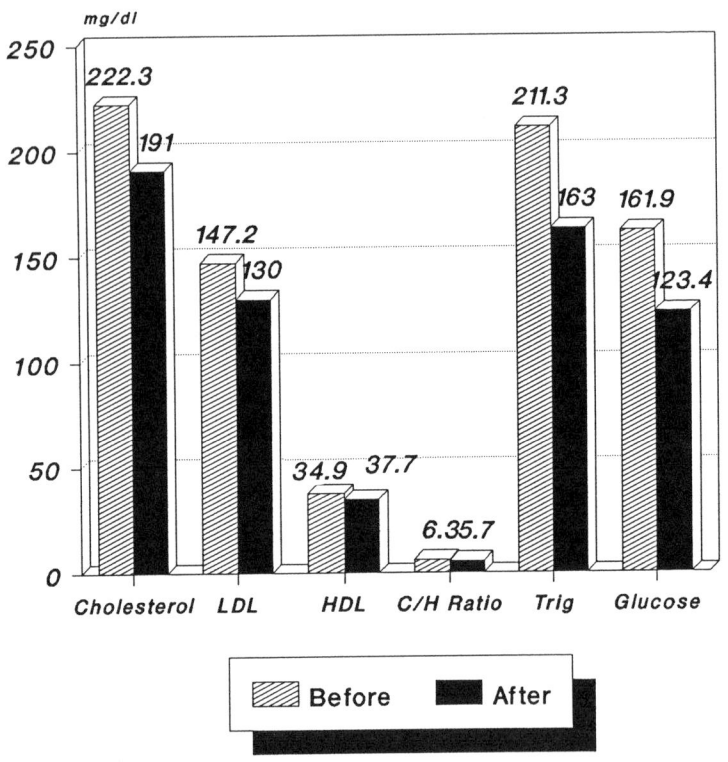

3. Cholesterol

Cholesterol is a waxy substance that deposits in arteries and causes heart attacks and strokes. These are the number 1 and number 3 killers of Hawaiians *(see graph on page 68)*. Cholesterol is found only in animal-type foods *(beef, pork, chicken, eggs, dairy, etc.)* and is not found in any plant type foods *(grains, fruits, vegetables, seaweed, etc.)*. Your cholesterol should be no higher than 200 mg/dl and is better if it is around 150 to 160 mg/dl. For every 1% you decrease your cholesterol, you decrease your heart attack risk by 2% until you get down to 150 mg/dl at which point your heart attack risk is practically 0.

In the Wai'anae Diet Program, the average cholesterol decreased an average of 14% from 222 to 191. This means a reduction in heart attack risk of 28%.

4. Blood Sugar

Blood sugar control improved for all seven participants who had diabetes. This is especially important because Hawaiians die faster of diabetes than all races in the U.S. *(see chart)*. The average blood sugar fell from 161.9 mg/dl to 123.4 mg/dl. A normal blood sugar is no higher than 120 mg/dl. One individual who continued the program for over a year no longer needs any diabetes medication after being on 60 units of insulin 3 years before the program. Because of this effect on blood sugar, if you are on diabetes medication, it is very important that you see your physician before changing your diet significantly.

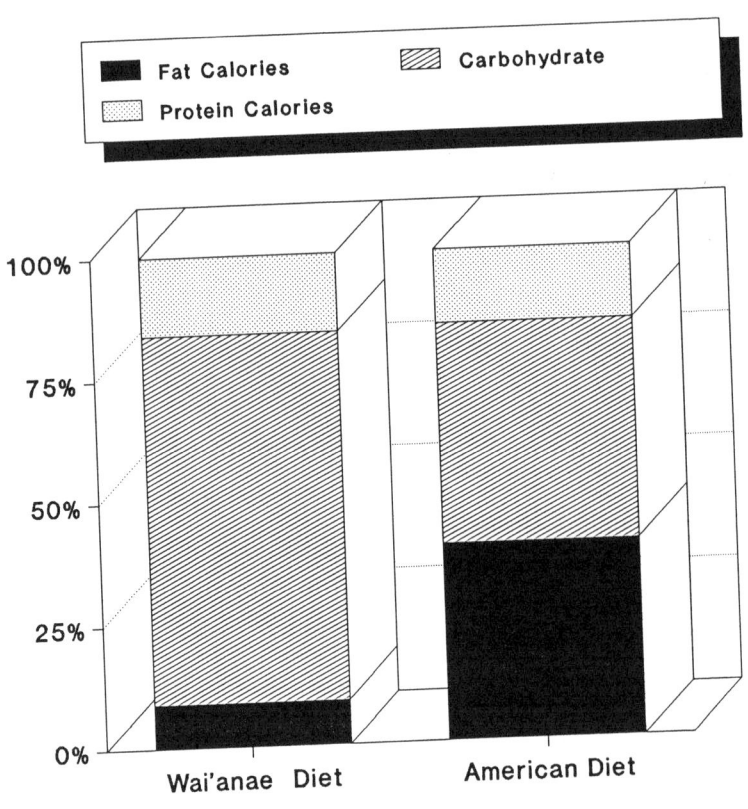

5. Composition of the Diet

The Wai'anae Diet was intended to reflect what Hawaiians ate in ancient times. It was very low in fat (7-12%), high in starches (75-80%) and moderate in protein (12-15%). This is in sharp contrast to the high fat Standard American Diet (S.A.D.). The S.A.D. has 400% more fat than the Hawaiian diet. Is it any wonder that high fat diets make high fat people?

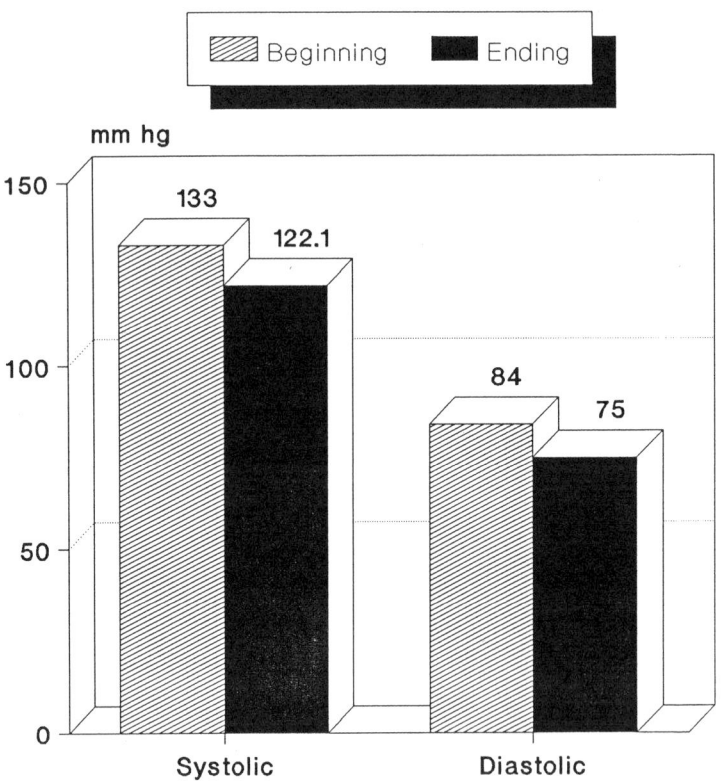

6. Blood Pressure

Blood pressure also improved significantly on the program. The average systolic blood pressure fell 9% and the diastolic pressure fell 11%. This is significant because high blood pressure increases the risk of heart attack and stroke. The diet may be so effective in lowering blood pressure that if you are on medication, it is especially important that you see your physician before drastically altering your diet.

COMMENTS FROM PROGRAM PARTICIPANTS

Mary Vea — The reason why I came to this diet was because I am a diabetic. It's a family history, and my family told me once I came on needles I will die on needles. When I met Ed Aikala one day at Diabetes Support Group, we were talking about the diet. He told me to have my doctor refer me to Dr. Shintani for the diet. So I did and when I got picked I was happy. Now being on the diet, I have lost weight and I got off insulin shots. For me I feel very strong, healthy, energetic, and I feel a great change in my body. I am very grateful and thankful to have a program like this and also to have people like Dr. Shintani, Helen, Midge, and Ed. But must of all we had each other to keep us from falling. Without us being a family, I couldn't have done it. I will give the project all my support and help. And I will let no one try to put this project down.

Joyce O'Brien — There was a time when my body was fairly attractive. Through the years I've used food as a stress relief . . . a comfort blanket. I **know** what is healthy foods and what is healthy amounts but the phrase "I'll start tomorrow" overshadowed my actions. "We want you around" my husband would often say. That statement, the vision of my family, my belief in the powers of traditional food and my personal, professional and community commitment brought me to this diet program determined to make a difference for myself, my health. It's been positive from the afternoon of day two. The first day and a half was a punishment for bad decisionmaking. Since then the bonding of **our** group, the confirmation of the qualities of **our** traditional foods, and the commitment of project staff has been emotionally and spiritually uplifting . . . words do this explanation an injustice. My family and I are extremely grateful for this experience.

Hoolehua Wright — Mahalo Ke Akua, Due to a broken ankle in 1987 and torn ligaments in 1991, I've been in so much pain in the early mornings, during physical activities and dancing the hula. Since I've been on the program, I've encountered no pain. The understanding of Lokahi, the help of Ke Akua, and the fine staff of this program have blessed me abundantly. Mahalo!

Aloha, My name is **Elmira Williams**. Since I've been on the Waianae diet program my blood pressure is stable. I am more alert mana, ano ano, aloha, kino. And for this I thank our lord in heaven, Dr. Shintani, Helen, Midge, Ed, and Robert Black Memorial Foundation — to the many other doctors and staff members of the Waianae Coast Comprehensive Health Center and especially to my family, who helped support me through this program.

Momi Kaehuaea — It was quite an honor to be picked as a participant for the Waianae Coast Diet Program. Results were awesome. My blood pressure is way down to below 116. I am doing things faster that I would drag through or dread to do before.

I find myself thinking clearer my outlook on life is better. And after checking with my other doctors they were amazed at my weight loss. I feel confident in myself. My family is amazed. I will continue this diet at home and intend to make it part of our daily meal.

I am exceedingly happy. Thank you Dr. Shintani, Helen, Midge and Ed.

Airleen Lucero — This Native Hawaiian Eating Program is great. I'm leaving the word diet out because it has a negative connotation. The program was an inspiration. It is truly a natural way of eating. I was full almost everyday. In fact, some days I could only eat half of my food.

I want to thank Dr. Shintani for his love, dedication and his vision that has made this all possible. Thanks to our cooks Mary, Bill, Midge and Coordinator Helen O'Connor for the beautiful meals.

The uniqueness of the program is, of course, the precious gems who have sparkled throughout the course of these few weeks. Mahalo to Ed Aikala for being an inspiration and an encourager to us all. The participants each gave of themselves and received in return health and life.

The guest speakers were also marvelous and helped to reinforce the Native Hawaiian concept of life and living. The spiritual connection to God, Aina and man makes this a beautiful and successful program. Aloha, Ke Akua.

Hugh Ko Mahoe — When I started my weight was 442 pounds and on Friday, 10-16-91 my weight is 426-1/2 pounds, three days before the end of the program.

This program has helped me lose some of my weight and I learned a lot about the Hawaiian culture and the spiritual part of our ancestors. I'm very thankful for being part of the project for it has made me feel good about myself, and I enjoy being with people that have weight problems too.

I hope Dr. Shintani can continue with more programs like this and that I can continue to be part of it.

Doreen Kolb-Latu — To the staff of the Waianae Diet Program, a special mahalo for helping me to understand the basic principles of health in a **positive** way. After many years of lectures and scare tactics by doctors, I only felt poor self-esteem and guilt. The Waianae Hawaiian Diet approach made me feel proud and culturally strong, as well as appreciating the **spiritual** foundations of food that gives Mana *(as opposed to "dead foods" that give pilikia/fats/sugar/processed junk food, etc.).* I am confident of continuing to lose weight and gain health, because I am "grounded" in culture. I appreciate especially, the role model of Ed, who **has** "walked in my shoes" and overcame the problem. If he could do it, I could too. Again, my thanks and I promise I will spread the word.

Jonnette Kaluhiokalani — I've been living on the Waianae Coast for 18 years with my husband and two son's. I'm overweight and have been feeling tired and my blood pressure was slightly high. Being on this program made me lose weight, my blood pressure has dropped, and I feel great! Reading and hearing about Ed Aikala's weight loss made me want to go on this program. I'm not cooking and buying as many junk foods like I used to. I'll be eating good nourishing food and do more exercise and will be taking good care of my body and health. I've been sharing this program with friends and family, and they would like to be on this program, too. I would like to thank the sponsors, staff and participants for all that was done for me. You all have been just great and I love you all!! Mahalo Nui Loa, Me Ke Aloha Pumehana.

Shawn Casuga — Hi, my name is Shawn and I am in the Waianae Diet Program because I want to lose weight so I can become better and can fit into better clothes. I hope that they like this comment about myself. Again I would like to thank Helen, Mary, Midge and Ed for helping me on this Diet Program. And again, that's all I have got to say.

Craig M. Kalawa — I love the food very much, but sometimes you wish you could eat Kalua pig and cabbage instead of fish all the time. I liked the taro and sweet potato, and most of all, the people who prepared them. It was wonderful how Midge, Helen, Terry and Ed could find the time to be so helpful to me and my family. Now me and Pua have to keep the faith, and try to continue on this natural but ono Hawaiian diet. Mahalo Noi Loa.

Puanani Kalawa — I feel the diet is a good diet. Sometimes it got hard to eat the taro, poi and sweet potato day after day. After awhile you wish for them to feed you more chicken than fish.

I'd like to thank Terry, Helen, Midge, Ed, and all of the participants who my family and I became close to during this period. Terry, Helen, Midge and Ed gave our family the tools to better health and now it is up to us to use them. Mahalo.

Ka'ula Kalawa *(2nd Grade)* — Ua maika'i ka diet. *(The diet was good.)* Ano maika'i ka Kalo ame ka 'uala. *(The taro and sweet potato was kind of good.)* Maika'i ka mai'a. *(The banana is good.)* Maika'i ka mea ai. *(The food is good.)* Maika'i lakou ka hana mea ai. *(The people who made the food is good.)* Maika'i ko'u kino. *(My body is good.)*

Shelly Enos — My experience with the Hawaiian Diet has been positive, completely painless and a learning experience that has extended into all aspects of my life – physical, emotional, spiritual, mental – every way. What most impressed me was what I learned about myself: my body responded so well, so quickly – weight went down, blood pressure went down, medication went down – and my ability to stay calm and focused under unusually severe stress was a new experience. And – I didn't cheat – not even once. I never knew I could be that strong.

My family has also benefited from this program because I am calmer, clearer, and healthier. I can handle, so they don't get my stress.

This Christmas I am giving my father and my aunts and cousins the Waianae Diet Book. I want them to be healthy and live longer along with me. If I have any regrets, its that I didn't go through this and learn early enough to save my uncle, who died at age 49. He would have loved this!!

Robert Donner, Sr. — When I came to this program on the advice from my doctor, my health condition was poor because I was very overweight and had high blood pressure, high cholesterol, and am a diabetic. I felt upset with my life and I have pains in my legs and arms and get short of breath real easy because of my glucose and high cholesterol.

Since I came to the Hawaiian diet my life has changed from bad to good because my insulin went from 40 units to 10 units in the morning and 20 units to 5 units in the evening.

I will continue the Hawaiian diet and do a lot of exercise so I can better myself. I feel grateful to have this opportunity because my health is getting better.

I feel very good about this program, and I wish this program can be continued to help other sickly people.

Peter Umi — Before I joined this program I was suffering from asthma, overweight and diabetes (oral insulin). The eating habits I have changed with this program I am going to continue. I have lost 20 pounds. I feel great right now. My asthma is very good. My wife likes me on this program and wants me to continue to lose weight and take care of my asthma and diabetes.

Aloha, I am **Myrtle Mokiao,** 72 years old and a Waianae Dieter Participant. Before this I suffered terribly. I couldn't walk, as I had a terrible wheezing problem and often out of breath. I have a bad heart, high blood pressure and diabetes.

Mahalo to you, I lost weight, my blood pressure is down and my diabetes is getting in control. I'm filled with energy, I walk great and I am very, very grateful to Ke Akua (God) for you.

You have once again given me **"A New Lease on Life."** Mahalo nui loa.

Eugene and Shawn Casuga —

Before the Program: I was tired more often, craving for sweets and fatty foods.

During the Program: When we were introduced to the program we were told that our food would consist of poi, taro, fish, sweet potato, fruits and luau leaves along with other foods — plus, Hawaiian tea and lots of water. At first I thought there would be no problem with the food. But I found out I had a hard time adjusting to no salt, no rice, gravies, and no fatty foods. One of my hardest meals that I had to adjust to was lunch at work because my fellow workers would bring out all the ono foods that I was so used to eating — but after explaining my situation to them — it become easier and easier to me. I then began to enjoy my food and the craving for other kinds of foods, began to leave me.

Ending of the Program: Now that I have adjusted to the foods and how I now feel and also think about foods — I realize it is the best thing I could have done for myself. I will not say, that I will not go back to my old ways of eating because it is possible. I will take it a day at a time and with the support of my family and friends that I have made here — we all can come out winners and set good examples for our extended families, friends and neighbors. What a contribution we can make to our community and country — a healthy one.

James N. (Kimo) Kaopuiki — This is the last day of our diet program. I'm in good health and know I will try to keep on doing what I have been taught. I have lost 15 pounds and 4 inches in my waist. The diet has helped my diabetes. My blood sugar used to be 400 and now it is 142. I have plenty of energy. At work I do a lot of heavy lifting and could only do a little bit. I used to get tired and short of breath. Now I can do a lot more. When I used to sit down and talk to somebody or when driving the car, I would fall asleep. I'm not doing that anymore — a good plus for me. I feel the change. Everybody at work is noticing.

God bless all the people that have helped with the program. Mahalo!

Aloha, **Paula-Ann Burgess** — Mahalo for this wonderful opportunity to bring wellness into my life. This experience is very difficult to put into words. My life prior to participating in this diet was a very average one. Like many of my ohana I allowed my body to go to waste including my intellectual capabilities and sense of self. Life that was controlled by the lure of unhealthy foods and lifestyle. After just one week on this diet I noticed changes, not only in weight but in my higher level of functioning at work which brought some very positive feedback from my supervisors. I also noticed changes in my attitude and feelings of control over what goes into my body. Culturally, it is good for me to know that the foods that nourished my ancestors nourishes me today. Through these foods, I am connected now. It is up to me and others to share this knowledge with our ohana and communities.

These past three weeks are the foundation for more changes, and I cannot express enough how appreciative I am for your generosity in helping to create this opportunity for all of us. Again, mahalo a nui loa.

Jennie Donner — Prior to the program my health condition was poor. I had high blood pressure, diabetes and overweight and cancer in the left breast. My doctor, Dr. Fred Dodge, told me about the program and how much it would help me and because it helped my husband in the past.

Prior to the program I had one thing in mind — to get off the insulin shots and better my health so I can keep up with my children, grandchildren and activities to come in the future.
This has all changed now. I am off insulin and down with my weight. I am happy about that. This affected my family because they are happy for me and hope their father would be in better health and off insulin too, like me.

I would try to stay on the diet and change my children's bad eating habits and to better their health for my grandchildren.

I am happy to stop taking insulin shots every morning and hope to stop taking high blood pressure pills. I know I can do it, with the help of God and the Hawaiian Diet Program we can all be healthy in mind, body, and spirit. Ancient Hawaiians had it, let's bring it back.

Jan Foster — Although I am the first non-Hawaiian to be on the program, I haven't had trouble getting used to the "real" food of the Hawaiian diet. The food except poi, fish and chicken was all new to me. The encouragement from everyone around me has helped me keep on going. I lost 15 pounds and I don't know how many inches. It has been an honor to feel part of the Hawaiian culture and to learn more from the inside out what it was to be Hawaiian before the western culture changed everything. I, too, now believe in the power of this food of this land to bring health and strength not only to the Hawaiian people but to all of us. My stamina/energy level is much higher. We are all glowing from the healthfulness of living this Hawaiian food program.

Without being "spoon-fed" to eat this low-fat, healthy diet, I don't know how I could have come to this point in my life where there is hope now that I can look the way God made me to look and live out the rest of my life in a healthy manner. I am so grateful to all of the staff — Dr. Shintani, Midge, Helen, Ed — and my fellow participants. This is a special time I will always treasure.

Rev. Leilani K. Sexton — When I tell people about the Wai'anae Diet Program, I tell them it helped me to choose my food a whole lot differently. You would have never seen fruits and vegetables on my plate! Red meat was my number 1 food. Red meat, rice and fried foods were a must. The only thing baked I liked was baked ham, baked pork roast and baked pork chops. And I had to have cakes and pies all the time. I always wanted to have the skin of the chicken.

When I first came off the diet I bought a box of chicken and I pulled all the skin off. I was proud of myself but couldn't throw the skin away. I knew I shouldn't fry it, so I baked it and ate it. But now because of the 21-day regime with special foods that I had to eat, because of my commitment to complete the program for my better health, I can now cook and eat skinless chicken, fish (white), vegetables and fruits without feeling guilty.

Lei wrote the Wai'anae Diet Lament - "When I Find Myself Ch Ch Ch Cheating."

Juanita Oclaray (7/1/92) — When you overload a circuit breaker – you have to reset it. If you have a surge protector for all your electronic gear and it trips off, you push a button to reset it. That's what the Wai'anae Diet did for me – reset my button! Ten years ago I weighed 100 pounds and only gained weight when I was pregnant. But after having my third child well into my 30's and poor eating habits *(7-11 chili-cheese nachos and a Big Gulp)*, I weighed 165 pounds in 1986. I lost about 15-20 pounds from 1986 to 1992. But it took the Wai'anae Diet to reset my way of thinking and my way of eating! I thought once it was over, I would have a hard time staying healthy and keeping the weight off, but it has allowed me to step back and make choices. I'm walking 14 miles a week and riding "Roller Blades" 1-2 times a week to keep in shape. It's great to feel good. And if this 100% haole can do it – so can you!

BEGINNINGS

The Waiʻanae Diet Program is just a beginning. We hope that it will be the start of positive changes in your life, and in the lives of those around you. We want to emphasize that the program is not just a diet of foods, but also of spiritual, mental, emotional, and physical growth as well. Use the recipes for mental, emotional, and spiritual growth every day along with the recipes for food. For now, traditional Hawaiian foods may be less available, so use the suggested substitute foods for variety. Traditional foods from other cultures also had great mana and healing power. As much as possible, involve your family, your ʻohana, because they will provide support. As the interest in traditional Hawaiian foods increases, more taro, poi, and other Hawaiian foods will be produced and become more available.

If you practice this program daily, your good health will improve, your family and others will take notice. If you share this program with your family and others, their health will also improve. This is the principle of "lōkahi" in action. You will become a teacher, and an important influence on the health of your family and the Hawaiian people. It is our hope that in this manner the health of our people will be restored. Me ke ʻonipaʻa.

BIBLIOGRAPHY

Blaisdell, Kekuni, "Historical and Cultural Aspects of Native Hawaiian Health," Social Process in Hawai'i, 32:1, University of Hawaii Press, Honolulu, Hawaii, 1989.

Center for Attitudinal Healing, "Principles of Attitudinal Healing," Tiburon, California.

Handy, E. S. Craighill, *Ancient Hawaiian Civilization*, revised edition, Charles E. Tuttle Co., Rutland, Vermont, 1981.

Malo, David, *Hawaiian Antiquities* (Mo'olelo Hawai'i) – Translated from Hawaiian by Dr. Nathaniel D. Emerson, Bernice P. Bishop Museum, Honolulu, Hawaii, 1951, reprinted 1987.

Nordyke, Eleanor C., *The Peopling of Hawaii*, 2d edition, University of Hawaii Press, Honolulu, Hawaii, 1989.

The 'Opelu Project Inc., *From Then to Now, A Manual for Doing Things Hawaiian Style*, Wai'anae, Hawaii.

Shintani, T.T. et al., "Obesity and cardiovascular risk intervention through the ad libitum feeding of traditional Hawaiian diet," Am J Clin Nutr 1991:53:1647S-51S.

Snow, Charles E., *Early Hawaiians*, University of Kentucky Press, Lexington, Kentucky, 1974.

Stanndard, David E., *Before the Horror*, Social Science Research Institute, Honolulu, Hawaii, 1989.

Van Dyke, Robert E., R. Rorvck, *Hawaiian Yesterdays*, Mutual Publishing Co., Honolulu, Hawaii, 1982.

Vaughn, Palani, *Na Leo I Ka Makani: Voices on the Wind*, Mutual Publishing and Edition Limited/Signature Publishing, Honolulu, Hawaii, 1987.

Waianae Coast Culture & Arts Society, Inc., *Ka Poe Kahiko O Waianae*, Top Gallant Publishing Co., Honolulu, Hawaii 1986.

NOTES

NOTES

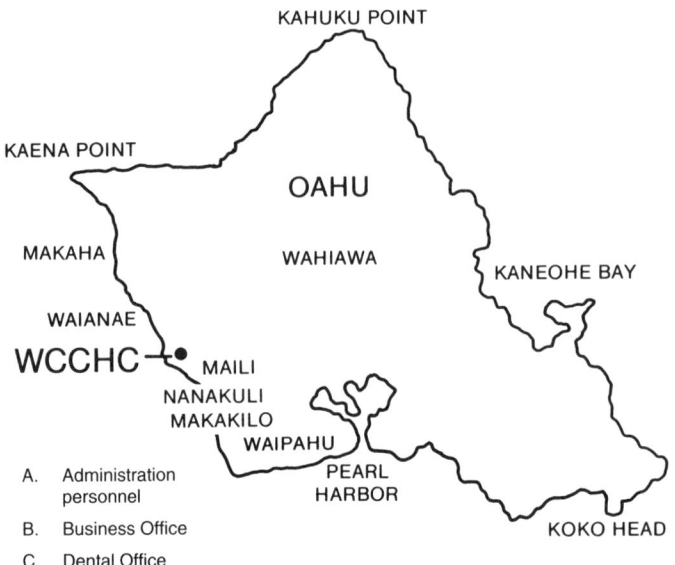

Waianae Coast Comprehensive Health Center

A. Administration personnel
B. Business Office
C. Dental Office
D. Medical Director's Office
   Home Health Services
   Medical Social Worker
E. Emergency Room
   Walk-in Family Medicine
   Laboratory
   X-ray
   Medical Records
F. Main Reception
   Pharmacy
G. Mauka Family Medicine
H. Makai Family Medicine
   (OLD FIRE STATION)
I. Adult Day Care
J. Health Education
   Nutrition/WIC
   Physical Therapy
   Occupational Therapy

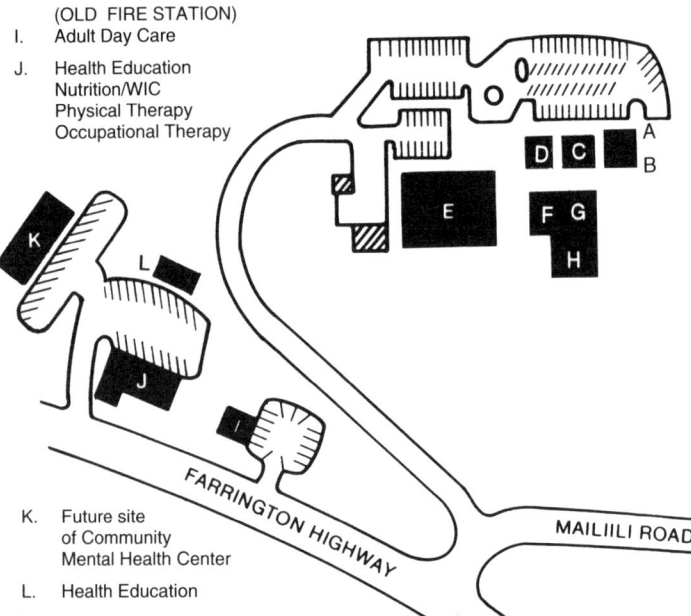

K. Future site of Community Mental Health Center
L. Health Education

Now Available

The Wai'anae Book of Hawaiian Health

The Wai'anae Diet Program Manual

This little book contains valuable insights for anyone interested in improving their health, following traditional practices of early Hawaiians.

The Wai'anae Diet Program demonstrated:

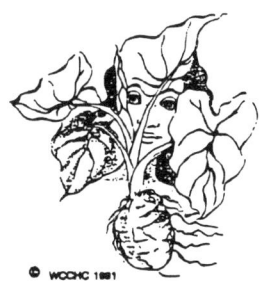

- Average weight loss in 21 days was 17.1 lbs.
- Cholesterol decreased 14%
- Blood Pressure decreased 10%
- Improved control of blood sugar
- Plenty to eat without counting calories

To order, fill out the form below and send $9.95 plus $1.75 *(postage and handling)* per book in check or money order to:

Wai'anae Diet Program
Waianae Coast Comprehensive Health Center
86-260 Farrington Highway
Wai'anae, Hawaii 96792-3199

Name _____

Address _____

City/State/Zip _____

Qty ____ Payment _____

(All proceeds go to support the Wai'anae Diet Program)

Now Available

The Wai'anae Book of Hawaiian Health

The Wai'anae Diet Program Manual

This little book contains valuable insights for anyone interested in improving their health, following traditional practices of early Hawaiians.

The Wai'anae Diet Program demonstrated:

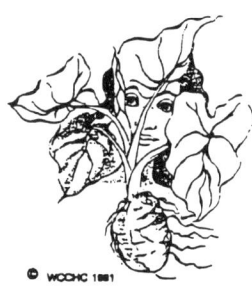

- Average weight loss in 21 days was 17.1 lbs.
- Cholesterol decreased 14%
- Blood Pressure decreased 10%
- Improved control of blood sugar
- Plenty to eat without counting calories

To order, fill out the form below and send $9.95 plus $1.75 *(postage and handling)* per book in check or money order to:

Wai'anae Diet Program
Waianae Coast Comprehensive Health Center
86-260 Farrington Highway
Wai'anae, Hawaii 96792-3199

Name _____

Address _____

City/State/Zip _____

Qty ____ Payment _____

(All proceeds go to support the Wai'anae Diet Program)